Baby Gone

Baby Gone

True New Zealand stories of infertility, miscarriage, stillbirth and infant loss

First published in
New Zealand in 2011 by
Hugs Press Limited
PO Box 27003
Wellington, New Zealand

www.babygone.com

Book trade distribution in New Zealand by Random House

Disclaimer
The views and experiences expressed in the stories in this book are provided by the general public and are therefore not necessarily those of New Zealand medical professionals and not-for-profit support organisations. Given this, the information within the book is not to be taken as medical advice. Jenny Douché has taken all reasonable care to ensure that the stories are free from errors and that they do not negatively implicate any person/s, profession or medical institution. To the extent permissible by law all liability (whether in negligence or otherwise) from the information in this book is disclaimed by Jenny Douché.

National Library of New Zealand Cataloguing-in-Publication Data
Douché, Jenny, 1971-
Baby Gone : True New Zealand stories of infertility, miscarriage, stillbirth and infant loss / Jenny Douché
ISBN 978-0-473-18046-1
Infertility – psychological aspects
Miscarriage – psychological aspects
Antenatal death – psychological aspects
Infant death – psychological aspects
Bereavement – psychological aspects
Pregnancy – psychological aspects
Dewey number: 306.9

Cover designed by Angela Vink
Cover photograph by Jenny Douché
Proofread by Vicki Andrews
Printed by Everbest Printing Co Limited

FOREWORD

There is nothing that can prepare you for the pain and grief of infertility or the loss of a much-longed-for baby.

My own story of loss began at a time when I felt my life was just about perfect. I was married to a wonderful man, living in a lovely country town and surrounded by friends and family. The business I had founded with my sister was growing rapidly and it seemed there was no stopping us. I felt the only thing missing in my life was a child.

Ours was the classic story of leaving things a little too late. At 38, a relatively short period of infertility ended in an ectopic pregnancy. Mercifully I was pregnant again soon after and at our 12-week scan it was revealed we were expecting not one but two beautiful little bundles.

We were ecstatic. Two for the price of one! We began the wonderful and exciting process of preparing for the arrival of our identical twins.

Our hopes and dreams were shattered by the event of our routine 20-week scan. It was then that we discovered the twins had a syndrome common to identical twins which, if left untreated, often results in the death of one or both twins.

Two days later we delivered our still born, still beautiful baby girls. The overwhelming amount of love and support from family, friends and work colleagues that followed was humbling and helpful, but I was not prepared for the depth of the grief and felt overwhelmed by it.

Over the long months after the loss of the twins I searched for a way to come to terms with what had happened and to find hope again. I discovered was that by far the most comforting and therapeutic form of dealing with the loss was talking about it with women who had experienced a similar loss.

Jenny Douché and I first met in 2003 when I interviewed her for a profile story in a women's magazine. At the time Jenny was busy publishing her hugely popular *Smarter than Jack* book series entertaining thousands of animal lovers around the world and raising a great deal of money for animal welfare.

Last year I heard from Jenny again. She'd heard about my loss and she had a new project, one that she thought would be close to my heart. As we sat down to discuss her plans for *Baby Gone*, we discovered that we'd lost our babies within days of each other and had both been blessed with healthy baby girls born just days apart the following year.

It was no surprise to discover that both Jenny and I felt the period after the loss of our babies was the darkest time of our lives, but in sharing our stories we felt an immediate, familiar and comforting solidarity.

I congratulate Jenny on the creation of this book, which I believe reflects a new awareness of the prevalence of infertility and baby loss in our society and a new willingness and freedom to talk about this important subject.

Despite the fact that these stories are written by women whose journeys, emotions and experiences will be different to yours and mine I am sure that, like me, you will find comfort in the similarities you'll discover in stories that make you stop and think *"I know exactly how that feels"* or *"thank goodness someone else thinks that way – I thought it was just me!"*

I hope the book will provide some of the answers you seek, and provide strength and resources for a future full of peace and hope for you and your family.

Catherine de Groot

INTRODUCTION

I suspect you're reading this book because, like me, your innocence has gone. You are now one of those people who know first-hand that things don't always go as planned. You have joined that special club, one that no one wants to join.

I'm sorry that you have a need to read *Baby Gone*, but I hope it will be of comfort, even if it is just in a small way.

I decided to compile this book after losing our son James in 2008. For ten days after he died I basically hid in my bedroom, not answering the phone and literally hiding when there was a knock at the door. I couldn't face seeing anyone except close family. I desperately wanted to read other people's stories of loss, and to feel like I wasn't going crazy.

Luckily my mother bought me some books, which I relished, however I really wanted to read stories that I could relate to, ones that were not sanitised. I wanted to know how it really was, and that I was not alone in my grief and all the intense and confusing feelings that it brings.

Alone I certainly wasn't. Did you know that in New Zealand about one in six couples of childbearing age are unable to conceive naturally, about one in four pregnancies end in miscarriage, and about 600 babies are either stillborn or die soon after birth each year? Add to this the dozens of small children who die accidentally or through illness. The impact of the loss of these innocent lives is immense.

About three months after James was born I created the idea for *Baby Gone*. But it was too soon to do it. Emotionally I was in a dark place, where I remained for a long time. I wasn't in a position to put my heart and soul into the detailed and emotionally demanding process of publishing a book. Two years later I was ready.

The stories in the book are from people throughout New Zealand. In September 2010 I put the word out and asked for submissions. Guidelines were supplied, with emphasis placed on wanting stories about the emotional side of the journey. I received over 100. What a difficult task it was selecting the best ones for publication. Every person's story was so important, but in order to ensure that the book had the right emphasis and mix of situations, I had to make some difficult decisions.

I'm so grateful to all those who took the time to write and send their very personal stories to me. It was such a privilege to read people's innermost thoughts, and in some cases it was the first time these thoughts had been shared with anyone, ever. Thank you to the contributors and their family members for so openly sharing your journeys with me.

Prior to creating this book, in 2002, I created a series called *Smarter than Jack*. These books contained true stories about smart animals and raised over $440,000 for animal charities around the world, including about $110,000 for the Royal New Zealand SPCA. Apart from the financial benefits to the charities, the books also helped to increase awareness of animal intelligence, in many instances leading to a gradual improvement in animal welfare.

Baby Gone exists because I want to help those who are unable to conceive or who have lost a baby at any stage. But I also want to make people involved in the care of women and their families more aware of what it is really like to not have a much-wanted child. This will hopefully lead to a greater understanding of the emotional journey and will result in a more compassionate level of care.

Thank you to all who were involved in the creation of *Baby Gone*, including Angela Vink for designing the cover, Vicki Andrews for proof-reading and Catherine de Groot for generously donating over 1,000 books to the medical community and support groups throughout New Zealand.

Thanks also to the 'grandparents' and to my husband, Anton, for looking after my children Matthew and Sarah while I spent many many hours working away on my computer, and thanks to Vicki Culling.

After reading the stories in this book you may feel the need to talk to somebody. At the back I have provided contact information for organisations and individuals who can offer support for infertility, and during and following the loss of a baby.

Finally, if you're wondering why there is chocolate on the cover, it is because, to me, chocolate symbolises the solace that I found within support organisation Sands. Every month, almost without fail, I would go along to the monthly support group meetings – and eat lots of chocolate – and talk and cry lots too of course.

They understood. I belonged. It was just what I needed.

Jenny Douché

Contents

WAYS TO READ THIS BOOK

What a dilemma it was trying to work out the best way to categorise the stories in this book.

It was not a simple matter of putting the stories in chapters of infertility, miscarriage, stillbirth and infant death. So many people had stories that covered a multitude of types of loss, all equally as devastating, so which chapter would their story go in? I didn't want some types of loss to be seen as being worse than others either – we are all grieving for the same thing, the child or children who are not with us today.

I decided it was best to not have chapters and to order the stories in a way that gives the reader variety in terms of types of loss, but also, very importantly, variety of experiences living with infertility or following the death of a baby.

However, many of you, quite understandably, want to go straight to stories that are similar to yours. So to help with this, on the next page is another contents section with the stories grouped by subject.

Infertility

Miscarriage

Stillbirth

Infant loss

I just couldn't get to the surface

Ruth McKenzie

Prior to going into that ultrasound room there was sunshine in my life. Beautiful, glorious, warm sunshine and I was happy.

I remember looking at the ultrasound screen pleading for there to be a heartbeat and repeatedly asking *"is there a heartbeat, is there a heartbeat".* The sonographer's eyes said it all.

That day the thunderstorm rolled into my life and the beautiful warm sunshine was gone. Life as I knew it had changed. My hopes and dreams for the future had changed. I had changed.

From the moment I found out that our precious unborn child was gone I felt like I had been thrown overboard in the middle of the rough ocean. Life suddenly was cold, the skies became dark with thick heavy thunder-clouds and the rain just poured. I was alone, in the middle of this cold dark ocean, drowning in the grief.

The grief that I felt for my unborn child was so overwhelming and deep that it just kept pushing me further and further under the water. I just couldn't get to the surface to catch my breath – and when I did, grief was waiting for me ready to push me down again, further and further each time.

The grief I felt was so intense that it was suffocating me. It was constantly there. It sat on my shoulders like a heavy burden, it lingered in my thoughts and it pressed heavily on my heart. Grief played tricks on me – it made me believe that it was my fault; I had failed as a mother and I couldn't do the one thing that a mother does best and that is to protect her child.

Life became unbearably hard. I would walk around in a daze with a constant lump at the back of my throat and always on the brink of tears. I was so sad and lonely. No one understood. There were days that I would sob my heart out on the bathroom floor for hours and all my husband could do was hold me tight, rock me back and forth, and lovingly stroke my hair. Nothing he could say or do would take the pain away.

Apart from family and a couple of friends the rest of the world moved on and chose to avoid and ignore my grief. I wanted them to ask if I was okay, I wanted them to ask what I had called the baby, I wanted them to acknowledge my sadness and my loss, and most of all I wanted them to comfort me. But never once did they ask or offer that longed-for caring touch.

Days turned into weeks and weeks turned into months and slowly my heart began to heal. The changes at first were very subtle. The rain changed to drizzle, the thunderclouds changed to overcast skies and the rough seas changed to gentle swells; slowly the darkness began to lift and occasionally a ray of sunshine would peak through the clouds.

But most importantly, every time I made it to the surface I was able to keep my head above water for that much longer each time, and even though grief was still waiting for me at the surface I felt stronger and more courageous each time and started to fight back.

Suddenly one day out of the blue the darkness was gone. The water was gone. The rain was gone. The thunderclouds were gone. And I was surrounded by beautiful, glorious, warm sunshine.

It was then that I knew I would be okay. I had survived.

Six years, nine months and 21 days

Michelle Denholm

I've been struggling with unexplained infertility for six years, nine months and 21 days.

It's come as a huge shock to me, because generally I've always been able to get what I want in life. You know, that boy in high school, the fantastic job, the home I fell in love with, the handsome and funny husband, reasonably good looks, lots of friends, that sort of thing.

My husband and I met 16 years ago. And ironically we accidentally fell pregnant about a year and a bit into our relationship. At the time our relationship was really rocky. We were both living at home, both hugely in debt, and I was scared that having the baby would break us up because of the strain of being young parents, and then I would be a solo mum. I was 22 at the time and he was 25. Not as young as some I know, but it was so important to me that if I were to bring a child into our world it would have a secure family. I felt insecure within the relationship.

I guess what I'm trying to say is that I made the decision to terminate. My husband (well boyfriend back then), was supportive of whatever decision I made. He actually did want to have the baby and his family was really supportive as well. But I was so staunch about raising a child in an emotionally and financially secure family environment. I wanted to have a good life for my child and me. I didn't want to be struggling on the bones of my ass for the rest of my life.

Skip ahead to today and our relationship is the strongest it's ever been because of our shared grief and broken dream of not having a family.

We've tried everything. Two rounds of IVF (in vitro fertilisation). The first round nothing, the second round a pregnancy but a miscarriage at six weeks. I produce quality A1 grade eggs and my husband's sperm was perfect. They fertilised our eggs with a combination of ICSI (intra-cytoplasmic sperm injection) and IVF on the first round and then ICSI all the way on the second round.

We've tried IUI (intrauterine insemination) with no result. We also tried Lipiodol, acupuncture, naturopathy, Ayurverdic medicine, massage, energy healing, hypnotherapy, eating no wheat and dairy, standing on my head, lying in bed after sex for 30 minutes, no alcohol, lots of alcohol, changing my cleaning products, vitamins, herbs, meditation, yoga, sleeping with a crystal on my tummy, praying, affirmations, writing letters to God and my guardian angels, crying, stamping my feet, threatening suicide, threatening to leave my husband. Of course the latter two have been threats to God and no one else.

I've had so many investigations and operations, I've actually discovered a liking for the drugs! Well, the ones that put you to sleep anyway. I've had a gazillion blood tests and the only thing that remotely gave an explanation is that my anticardiolipins were a little high (which makes your blood thicker than normal). I took baby aspirin for a year and have been on folic acid for the last six!

It's been a tough journey. In fact, last November I seemed to have reached my limit and was on the verge of antidepressants. Things were just so bad and I was so unhappy all the time. My marriage was on the brink because of my awful behaviour. I guess I just had to realise that I wasn't coping, and I was grieving. I had to stop pretending that everything was okay. I had to stop putting on the happy face and stop being extra-excited for friends and family when they announced their pregnancies. And I had to wake up to the reality that it may not happen for me in this lifetime. And that it hurts. It's the worst experience I have had in my life, aside from my mum dying.

It's an experience I wouldn't wish on my worst enemy. It's absolutely devastating to your spirit and your soul. It changes you. It's humbled me. It's brought me to my knees, literally.

I forgive those people (for the most part anyway) who make insensitive comments such as *"are you sure your husband's not shooting blanks"* ha ha ha, they laugh. Usually it's men who make that remark. Or *"just relax and it'll happen"*. In fact I'm so OVER hearing that part about relaxing. People can be thoughtless.

One instance in particular. When a friend was asked the question if she was going to have any more children, she replied *"no I'm not having any more kids, I'm too old"*. She's one year older than me, and that was two years ago. Am I being too sensitive? Do I read too much into what people say? Do I take what they say as a personal swipe at my childlessness? Probably. But the reality is that I *am* sensitive about this topic.

But people who haven't been through conception difficulties have no idea about what we go through. How can I expect them to know how I feel when they haven't had that life experience? So for this reason I do try hard not to focus on other people's comments.

I guess I am what you call a Type A personality. I do find it hard to relax because I like everything to be perfect. I set extremely high expectations of myself and others. I have often wondered if this is a common thread for women who are struggling to conceive because we put so much pressure on ourselves. I like the house to be in perfect order before I sit down to 'relax'. I'm getting better in my old age … I think.

I'm now 36. And people tell me *"oh but you're still young"*. Yeah but my dream was to get married and have kids. My dream was that my children would be around the same age as my nephews and nieces; they would grow up together, play together and be great mates. My dream was that I would still look young in family photos with my children. My dream was that we would have a family of our own.

More than anything, I've felt like a failure as a woman, as a wife and as a human being. It's been a cold hard slap in the face to me. Is it an ego thing, this quest to have biological children of our own? I'm open to adoption, but my husband is dragging his feet. Whenever I bring up the topic he says *"you've got to have faith, it's going to happen for us"*. I love that he is so positive, but my faith has dwindled down to near zero.

I can honestly say though that at the moment I am in a good place. Since last November I have been in the process of making peace with the situation. I constantly affirm *"in perfect trust I surrender to divine timing"* (this does bring me a degree of peace). I refuse to do another IVF. After both rounds I broke out in a full body rash, not to mention the absolute devastation of doing all that shit and it didn't work. I refuse to pay all that money and not be guaranteed a baby. I would dearly love to help a child who really needs it.

I'm over the specialists who pooh-pooh my suggestions of considering an endometrial biopsy and the role that immunity plays in conceiving. New Zealand has to get with the rest of the world and seriously consider the autoimmune system and the role it plays in conception. The specialists are all admitting that natural conception rates are declining, and there has to be a reason. Money needs to be invested into finding out why!

I've been ridiculed by the first specialist I saw for charting my temperature and giving him my own opinion of a possible short luteal phase.

In fact I think his exact words were *"you don't need to be bothered with all that mumbo-jumbo"*. (About the temperature charting I mean.)

I've scanned the internet a thousand times to try and find out what's wrong with me.

Personally, I wonder about our world. The stress levels, the shit in our food, the pollution, the pressure to look a certain way, to have certain things, to be Mr and Mrs Perfect. I fantasise about a simple life. Living rurally on a few lush acres with a gorgeous brand new contemporary home with an organic vege garden, and I work three days a week, 10–2am. And all my friends and family live rurally too on their acreages, and we get together on Saturdays to swap foods from our gardens, whilst our kids play and we drink wine. Us girls all look younger than we are because we eat organically and breathe the fresh country air and our husbands are hot, funny and strong. Oh and we all have money trees growing in our backyards too so money isn't a problem.

I guess I want it all. And I always have. Is that too much to ask? I don't think so.

I've come to the conclusion that, in this lifetime anyway, I might not be a mum. But in my past and certainly future lifetimes, I was and will be a mum. I believe we are spiritual beings having a human experience. I look for the lesson in every experience, and so far I believe my lesson is to let go and trust. And whilst it's painful not getting what I want, it is fantastic having sleep-ins, going on tropical holidays, being able to afford $700 boots and having the time to build an amazing relationship with my husband. We girls have to look at the positives.

Good luck my darlings.

So brave and always kept her smile

Angela Schleif

On 9 November after a very normal pregnancy and a C-section birth (due to the breech position), our first child was born. A beautiful little girl, perfect in every single way, we named her Abby. I fell in love with her instantly; it was a different kind of love, one that I had never felt before – something I think only a parent can feel for their child.

Our first year was normal, wonderful and uneventful. Abby was a very healthy child, with only one visit to the doctor for normal baby stuff. She was such a happy wee girl, always smiling and trying to get everyone's attention so she could give them a big cheeky grin. She brought so much joy to our lives. I felt like this was what I was made to do, be Abby's mum. We had so much fun together and I utterly delighted in her – our time together was so special.

Towards the end of her first year we noticed she was quite small for her age and was a later crawler than the other kids. We were told that all kids are different and that they develop and grow at different rates. She looked healthy and had a bright personality – we really didn't worry too much at her being a little bit behind.

We thankfully threw her a big first birthday party with all her friends. She had a great time being the centre of attention and nibbling on fairy bread. We have lots of photos (again thankfully) of this special day for her and us, which turned out to be her one and only birthday.

Two weeks later at 11pm we found her having what looked like a small seizure in her left hand. It turned out to be a massive seizure; they wouldn't stop even after huge adult doses of anti-seizure drugs – and they went all through the night. They finally stopped about 6am after she was induced into a coma in ICU (intensive care unit).

Our world was completely turned upside down. To go through that and see your baby lying in an ICU ward in a coma, with all those horrid tubes – so vulnerable. There was nothing I could do but pray. It was terrible not knowing what was happening or what the outcome might be.

We feared her brain might be damaged, or that she may not use the left side of her body properly again. Nothing in this world could have prepared us for the next eight months of tests, exploratory operations, drugs, on-going seizures, constant vomiting and adverse reactions to the myriad of drugs that doctors tried to control her seizures. She had weeks of staying in hospital being poked and prodded, and feeling dreadful, but still she was so brave and always kept her smile. I was such a proud mum!

Eight months after she had her first seizure she was released from her suffering and went to heaven. My husband and I were so thankful to be there to say goodbye and tell her how much we loved her as she left this cruel world.

I held her limp body wrapped around me, and sang her all her favourite bedtime songs over and over. I told her many things as she lay dead in my arms, there was so much I wanted her to know, so much that I needed to tell her. I had a lifetime of mother and daughter conversations that she needed to hear and this was it, my last chance – but really it was too late. My brain just couldn't process it, my baby was gone.

Finally after several hours I said goodbye and that I would see her in heaven someday, that she had my blessing to go. That was the last time I ever held her in my arms.

Life has never been the same since that horrid night. I'd been so strong while she was sick, but now my life felt sucked dry – there really wasn't much left. Initially, for the first three months, it was total shock and disbelief – I was in my own very small world and honestly didn't know whether I was coming or going.

After the birth of our son Kody, three months after Abby died, the reality kicked in and that's when I started to feel like I was going crazy. Abby was really gone and this new baby wasn't her, she wasn't coming back ever.

For many months after Abby died I felt tired and had no energy. It took a huge amount of work to be around people and to act like everything was okay when in fact it wasn't. I was consumed by Abby, her death, my sadness, and this huge loss. I didn't spend a lot of time with friends, I just wanted to be alone and to feel sad – to look sad. It took less effort and I could cry whenever I felt like it – which was often! I also felt sad for my life – it was all messed up, this was not how it was meant to go. I was never going to get over this, not in a million years!

I started to realise I felt better if I was a little hungry all the time, because the mild discomfort in my belly actually lessened the constant pain in my chest/heart. I felt crazy at times, I felt I was going mad.

Sometimes I'd feel like I'd left Abby somewhere or forgotten to pick her up and have a little panic – until reality kicked in and that was even worse. I called Kody 'Abby', and got mixed up with 'he' and 'she' all the time. I was often convinced that both my kids were sleeping peacefully in the house when it was quiet. It felt good to dream even though it was brief!

I just wanted her back! My body ached to hold her, she had spent so much time in my arms. I was constantly filled with sadness. My health suffered, my nerves were shot. I didn't care about life, was just waiting for it to be over – wondered how I could ever really enjoy life again, after what I had been through. I kept going over her treatments, seeing her face during all those tests – when she cried. All those nights in hospital with broken sleep, as she needed monitoring throughout the night. Me holding her and comforting her – trying to make it all okay when it wasn't. Thinking about her last few days – reliving them over and over.

I had guilt, sometimes I wasn't even sure what about, just everything. I should have been able to make it better for her. I made her who she was, I was so sorry I had not created her with perfect health. I told her I was sorry many times – alive and dead.

Abby's things were throughout our house, I couldn't let her go. I wanted to mother her, do anything big or small to feel like I was still looking after her. I remember wanting to see her in her grave, dig her up – I didn't care in the slightest what she would look like. She was my baby girl – I was her mummy! She was mine, I should have her, I should be able to see her whenever I pleased. It was so unfair that she should be so out of reach to me. I'd lost my place in the world, the person I used to be had gone. I wanted to be normal again, to be okay, not so consumed. Friends were distancing themselves and I didn't have the energy to pull them back.

It felt good to talk about her, I wanted to talk about her all the time. But it just felt weird because everyone looked so uncomfortable at the mention of her name. There weren't many brave enough to be the first to utter her name in a conversation but I wished there were, even now. Nobody could understand even for a second, except maybe my husband – but it wasn't easy for him to talk about her all the time either. It was hard on our marriage, men deal with things so differently and we had very different styles of grieving.

Some days I'd start to feel better – but then that would make me feel guilty and miserable. I dreaded the one-year anniversary of her death – it made me feel so sad that I would never be in the year that she had been alive again. It just felt like I relived the lead-up to her death – in real time – so slowly, one event at a time as that awful day grew closer.

After the one-year anniversary, I was so relieved and realised it wasn't actually anywhere near as bad as I thought it would be. I have now survived that anniversary three times and it does get a little easier as each year passes. On a daily basis I am still filled with deep sadness that she is gone. It makes me cry from time to time that she's not here and I still sometimes can't believe it's true. But she lives on in my heart and I feel very close to her. That closeness hasn't faded at all, unlike the awful memories which are becoming less vivid and poisonous with time.

I know that one day I will see her in heaven, that beautiful smile, and it will be like no time at all has passed; she will be happy once again and have a perfect healthy body! I am now 16 weeks pregnant with a healthy baby girl and am absolutely over the moon. Abby and Kody will have a new baby sister.

This new baby won't fix me

Laura Hurley-Berry

I can't believe how much my life has changed in one short year, how a life so short yet mammoth could do this. I could never have imagined my new reality would involve losing my firstborn at 38 weeks to stillbirth and then being left to carry on. Most of the time I don't know whether to be sad or angry.

Ever since losing her I have longed to be pregnant again and prove not only to the world but to myself that I can have a healthy baby. Now that I am – following another loss, a missed miscarriage at nine weeks – all I want is for someone to tell me everything will be okay this time. I want them to say with some authority that I will get to bring home a healthy, breathing, pooing, weeing and screaming baby this time round, but no one can say this with the authority I need.

I live in constant fear that this baby will stop moving and I'll hear those horrible words again, *"I'm sorry, there's no heartbeat"*. I often marvel that I survived the first time, without even entertaining a second; that I have continued to survive each day without losing my mind. Initially I convinced myself that I would be cured of the constant and all-consuming fear once I could feel this new baby move and kick, but this has brought a whole new level of anxiety to the table.

It is quite usual for me to feel a rising panic after not feeling the movement for as short a time as ten minutes or to wake in a panic, frantic for the baby to show me it's alive. I try to convince myself that by paying attention to the kicking and the choices I make, I have control – but in reality I am merely a passenger on this journey, hoping for the best outcome. I try not to burden others with these thoughts, I keep them inside. I can't bring myself to go to the hospital if I'm worried for fear they'll deliver bad news. Instead I sit alone hoping and willing the baby to move and planning another funeral until it obliges; then I can carry on, albeit for a short time.

I'm caught between wanting time to stand still in the moment when my daughter was the centre of my physical world and wanting to fast-forward to a time when I actually have a living child – if that time exists. I see-saw between pure excitement for this new baby and devastating grief and longing for my daughter who isn't here.

Thoughts of losing another baby are never far from my consciousness. What if I never get a living child? What sort of mother does that make me? What sort of woman does that make me? Failing at the very essence of what it means to be a mother, a woman. Disappointing my husband, my family and my plans for the future.

I look around at those who still have that unconditional faith in life and I feel sick to my stomach. I envy their naivety and I envy their confidence that everything will be okay. Sometimes I even envy their lives. I cling to the remnants of hope; however, much of this was unfortunately lost along with my daughter. Hearing of others' pregnancies brings on these symptoms of physical sickness, which is beyond my control. It's as though my brain doesn't register this baby, only that yet another couple will get a living baby before we do.

It's amazing how much detail I remember after losing my daughter despite the whole situation being a blur: kind words that were spoken, the inappropriate and hurtful words unleashed, the actions of some, the inactions of others. These are forever etched in the essence of who I am and I'm sure will manifest themselves once this baby is born, much to the surprise and possible distress of those involved. I can't and won't apologise for this, I see it as a way of protecting my daughter's memory and attempting to be the parent that I feel I am but few acknowledge. A similar scenario is unfolding with this pregnancy: comments and actions by family, friends and health professionals may seem unimportant to the individuals but remain etched and replay in my mind constantly. A split second feels like an eternity to me, but I know from the past that in a moment your world can be changed forever.

At this point of this pregnancy, I can no longer keep my new baby a secret; as such I have to deal with increasingly difficult scenarios. It's hard to decide which is more difficult. Strangers who don't know about my daughter, who feel obliged to comment on my pregnancy and the sleepless nights ahead – can't they read the look on my face, don't they realise losing a baby leads to sleepless nights too? Or the people who 'know' and who treat me like an outcast, who assume I can no longer cope with normal social interaction, people who I used to call friends, that don't mention my daughter or this pregnancy and give me a look of pity at every opportunity.

I don't really fit in anywhere, I'm not a first-time mum but I'm not a practising one either. Even the health professionals involved in this pregnancy don't really know where I fit in; I feel like I am the first and only mother to lose a baby and then decide to tread the lonely path of trying again.

I'm asked questions about birth and breastfeeding but I can't even bring myself to that point. I live day by day, sometimes moment by moment. Small activities like thinking of names and baby gear sap my energy, all I can think is that dead babies don't need anything except a coffin. All these 'details' just seem unimportant, until this baby is here safely.

I'm made to feel abnormal, detached for behaving this way, but I know everything is a coping strategy – a way of getting through the long days and nights ahead.

I know this new baby won't fix me, I'm broken and part of me will remain that way. In fact to start with, if this baby does live I think it will high-light all the beautiful moments I missed out on with my daughter – a mixed blessing I guess.

I'll never know what sort of mother I would have been, and I'm too uncertain regarding the final weeks of this pregnancy to plan what sort of mother I will be this time, for fear of losing more of myself should this baby join its big sister.

I finally sobbed in grief

Anonymous

When I was growing up it was quite acceptable to marry early. Because of our family circumstances – a solo parent and three children (unusual then) trying to survive on a woman's low wage and my junior female's income – my mother encouraged me to marry so at 17, with a certain amount of desperation and innocence, I did, not choosing wisely, and violence became part of my life.

Ignorance about pregnancy precautions was fairly universal and I was soon 'in the family way'. After a particularly bad night of marital disruption when I was about 19 weeks along, I began to bleed. I'd had to quit work as I vomited constantly the whole pregnancy and had become very frail and quite depressed, so this seemed like just another problem I did not feel up to handling, especially not that morning. In my ignorance I thought *"it will go away after a while"* or (dramatically) *"maybe I'll bleed to death"* although I don't think I really believed that, but I didn't care too much one way or the other.

Life didn't seem worth living anyway and I was still in shock about what was happening and also about how my gentle, polite, caring husband had changed once I became his wife.

I had never heard of miscarriage and it wasn't until my mother eventually came to see me that I found out what was happening. She'd had several herself, although I now think some might have been abortions, given what I found out later.

No one went to a doctor unless they absolutely needed to, and my husband wasn't about to take me to the doctor with bruises still showing. So I went along by myself and the doctor inspected what I had passed in the night (chambers were used frequently then – especially with outside toilets) and said to me *"you were carrying twins"*.

I wandered around for days afterwards, isolated from everyone (courtesy of my husband), in a semi-dazed state. I kept thinking about the two little babies, feeling guilty, but in a way I was glad they hadn't been born into our circumstances.

Because I was an outpatient at the hospital, I rang from a public phone box (not many people had phones at home) to cancel my next appointment and explain what had happened. They were very quick to end the conversation and in fact said quite shortly I hadn't needed to ring at all!

I remember afterwards standing outside the phone box in the shopping centre, facing the road, with my hand across my face to avoid oncoming traffic seeing me quietly crying, before pulling myself together enough to face people and walk back home on the busy footpath. Once home I wandered around the garden trying to understand my emotions. I didn't even associate the word 'grief' with what I was feeling.

When I started a job again a few weeks later, I mentioned my miscarriage to a woman colleague. She thought it was no big deal and expected me to just get on with life. So I did and never mentioned my loss again – to anyone. I didn't talk about it again until years later when I became a member of a miscarriage group, but even then I minimised it as others seemed so much more distraught than me with more recent traumas.

For years it was a vague part of that life I didn't really want to remember once I was out of it. I went on to have children, all with the constant vomiting, with a new partner who became my husband. However, I also lost our first pregnancy, at about the same three-month time frame as previously. One night when we were nearly asleep we had both felt the tug in my stomach. I didn't really get that it was the beginning of another miscarriage, although he may have. I woke about an hour later and felt the strong urge to go to the toilet and couldn't believe how fast everything happened.

I sat on the edge of the bath still half-asleep shaking in shock for a while afterwards with towels soaking up the residual blood, not wanting to go and wake my partner because he was probably going to be more upset than me. And he was. I felt so dreadful for him and guilty for letting him down. We just held each other for ages before talking about going to hospital. He was very good with the physical side of the miscarriage – much better than me, being off a farm – and had no problem dealing with all the blood.

After having a D&C (dilatation and curettage), I went for a six-week check-up with a local doctor that I had never met before as we were new to the area. When the doctor found out that my partner and I were not married, he angrily accused me of aborting myself. This was prior to the physical examination. I sat opposite him, so angry at being accused of something I would never do, but which I felt guilty about anyway. I kept looking at the paper knife on his desk. Part-way through his moral/religious lecture I just got up and walked out, just in case I was tempted to use it. I was distraught and angry.

The memories of my losses are still with me today as clearly as when they happened.

Many years later, and I'm talking 40 years here, a visiting midwife friend who knew my history used the bathroom and commented on the two tiny, beautifully dressed dolls with long curly hair that sat on a small shelf that she saw in there. I was attracted to the dolls because there was a familiarity about them, partly their hair which was similar to my own when I was little. I was not particularly vain and I'd never really been a doll person so I surprised myself that I had bought them, which I had done separately.

I looked at the dolls every day for ages just admiring them until the friend's visit when she said *"I see you have two tiny dolls as a reminder of your lost twins"*. I suppressed the shock and tears till she had gone, and then just sat in my lounge finally sobbing in grief for all my little lost babies.

We were not permitted to grieve

Gaye

Michael died in September 1967. He was too young to die, and unfortunately too young to live; he came after only four months of gestation.

We were devastated. My husband and I had tried for several months to conceive, and when we finally did we were overjoyed. Our joy turned to sorrow and pain. At the hospital, the nurse told me that sometimes this happened with a first baby, and having a D&C (dilatation and curettage) often 'fixed' it. We were not permitted to mourn or grieve.

Others were not so caring; some were very callous.

"Well, it wasn't really a baby, only a foetus."

So when does the foetus you conceive become a baby? To us, he was always a baby. We prepared for his arrival until there was to be no arrival of a live baby.

"Never mind, you can have another one."

If I said that to someone whose son was killed in a car crash, how would they feel?

But we wanted this one, as well as any others we may conceive. There were no answers then, and very likely none now for lots of situations. What people did not realise is that losing a baby is a death in the family, but we were not permitted to mourn or grieve.

It took a long time to let go.

A year later we welcomed the arrival of a healthy little girl and that heartache was eased, but we never forgot; how can you forget the child you have conceived with love and joy?

Another year later, our next baby, Simon, died. Why? No one had answers.

The callous people said,

"Never mind – you have a lovely baby girl …"

Although it was comforting to hold her in my arms and love her, it did not change the fact that another son had died inexplicably.

Another year went by, and Luke suffered the same fate, and this time I was really ill. I bled all night before the doctor came, and I was some time in hospital needing a blood transfusion to go along with all the misery.

"Never mind – you have a lovely little girl …"

But we had three sons who had died …

My husband was getting rather stressed out over this, especially watching me nearly bleed to death, and decided that we should not try again. It was too distressing for him and for me.

But …

The desire to give birth is incredibly strong, and three years and two miscarriages after our first little girl, we had another healthy little girl without any trouble at all – apart from my father dying round about the time I had been prone to miscarry. But this little girl was determined and tenacious, and she arrived, healthy, whole and 16 days overdue!

Many years later, I was talking with a nursing friend about it and told her that I had always considered it was blood incompatibility – which my doctor did not accept; my husband and I are the same blood group, but he is Rh- and I am Rh+. He said it was the other way around, and that blue babies now have a much better chance of survival with pre-birth blood transfusions, and a vaccine that has now been created. I was cross about that, grumping to my husband that one day some professor of medicine would get the Nobel Prize for medicine by proving my theory.

My nursing friend told me I was right. I was astounded to have some-one agree with me! Turns out she was from a medical family: doctors, lab technicians, surgeons, you name it. An aunt who had the same problem thought the same thing – being a lab technician, she had the ability to test it out and found it to be so – and the fact that both our daughters have my blood grouping confirms for us that unanswered question of why we lost so many sons.

There are still so few answers to many things in the world of medicine. When people pat you on the head and say *"never mind"*, they are not help-ing one bit. We do mind, and mind with great hurt.

Unfortunately, both our daughters have also lost a child, but knowing that their mum and dad have been down that road made it easier for them to handle it.

The grief of expectations dying

Frank Rolfe

My name is Frank and this is my story about our son Eli who was stillborn on 4 September 1994. He died inside his mum the day before.

My wife has five children to a previous marriage: four healthy and one miscarriage.

We decided to have a baby, which my wife very much wanted to give me as it would be my first child. She fell pregnant fairly quickly. We had a bit of a scare at the first scan at around 18 weeks. After the scan the specialist called and said they couldn't see the baby's ribcage properly, and that it could be a sign that something was wrong. We had to wait another week for a scan to find out that all was okay. That was a long week, but I didn't feel too worried as I was sure that I had seen the ribcage during the first scan.

So the pregnancy went on, with baby talk and various plans made. We were 99% sure that the baby was a boy as we had watched those scans real close. The thought of having the family name carry on gave me a neat feeling.

We had been getting our ten kicks a day and all seemed okay. There was nothing to point to what might be coming.

On Saturday we went to my cousin's baby's christening. It was good to talk with the family about our upcoming delivery. Then on the Saturday night my wife had a cold feeling. We talked about calling the midwife and decided to leave the call until the morning.

Sunday was Father's Day. We called the midwife, who came to examine my wife. She said we needed to go to the hospital. I was unaware at this stage that she couldn't pick up a heartbeat on her little monitor. It usually sounded like galloping horses to me. It was about 9.30am.

I remember clearly stopping at the garage to check the car's tyre pressure and having to wait for a lady blowing up her bike tyre. I was excited at this stage and shared with the lady that we were going to the hospital to have our baby. I recall seeing a look of fear and worry on my wife's face as I got back into the car.

We went into a room and our midwife hooked up the big monitor. She got the doctor on call, who just happened to be our doctor. He couldn't pick up the baby's heartbeat and so went to get the specialist. My wife and I prayed.

It was now about 10.30am. The baby still wasn't moving and it was noticed that there was a big layer of fat on its tummy, which pointed to pregnancy diabetes.

We had questions to answer. Did we want to deliver now? Did we want to go home and let things happen naturally?

All I wanted was to do whatever my wife wanted, and so we had a natural delivery. They gave her medication to bring on labour, and then we had to just wait. To add to the goings-on, our friend was in labour at the same time. Her husband knew of our situation, but we kept the news from his wife until the next day. I had a big cry on his shoulder in the men's toilets in the maternity ward. That was one of the few safe moments where I could let go and just cry and yell or do whatever.

We had family, friends, midwives, doctors all at the delivery. It's a wonder we all fitted in the room. We all cheered my wife on. I can say, as a father, that being present during a natural birth is an amazing experience, even though our baby, a boy we called Eli, was not alive.

After the birth my wife's two young boys, aged six and eight, came to see their brother. Before seeing Eli, I took them to another room, got down to their level and explained that things had gone wrong.

Even 16 years on I can still recall every detail as if it has just happened.

When I brought my wife home the next day we just sat by the empty cot and cried. I was in protection mode for a while afterwards, mainly for my wife as she was having trouble facing day-to-day life and she had just had the physical trauma of delivering a baby. She had nothing to hold. Neither did I.

I took on all public duties like shopping and getting the photos developed. I had to stand in queues with new babies on mothers' shoulders facing me, cooing. It was very hard.

Through all of this we kept communicating. We made a decision early on that this wasn't going to drive us apart, as can often happen.

At night I would stay awake as long as I could so I'd be so tired that I'd just fall asleep, however I would wake up feeling worse than when I went to sleep. I have never experienced that feeling of intense grief before, although I have had people close to me die. Could it be the grief of expectations dying? You expect to bury people older than you, we bury our parents. Our children bury us, not the other way round. It goes against the natural.

We looked for answers but were given none. There were contributing factors, but no real reason. This is quite common, based on what we have heard from others who have gone through something similar.

Then came the decision, do we try again, can we try again? Well, medically we were able to. We were advised that as age was not really on my wife's side we needed to make our minds up soon, so we did.

Now, people may be creatures of habit or not, but the due date for our next son was one year to the day of Eli's birthday.

It was an exciting, nervous and well-monitored pregnancy, followed by a successful C-section delivery due to a true knot in his umbilical cord. The outcome could have been very different if we had had a natural delivery.

The loss of a child for me was not a natural process. I fought in my mind for a long while afterwards, researching facts, the autopsy results; nothing was abnormal, everything seemed fine, but there were some contributing factors. But no one could say what the cause was, and that was the biggest fight in myself, my attempt to justify why.

I've learnt a lot about women, pregnancy, the reproductive system, how common miscarriage is, stillbirth and newborn baby death rates. I used to be so blissfully unaware. I now know a lot more than the average man should ever know.

What could have helped me back then was having up-to-date information and support groups, like there are now. I am now part of a local Sands group and am on the national board. Where I can, I care for others who have joined the ranks of being a bereaved parent of a baby.

Eli changed my life. He made me look at what was really important. I changed careers. I followed my passion without fear, without drudgery. Eli has made me more caring, slightly tougher and definitely unafraid of what might come my way.

Thank you Son.

I remember her first and last kick

Anonymous

On 8 March 2010 I found out I was pregnant. I had taken my pregnancy test two weeks after I had conceived. I was raped on 19 February so the process of getting through the emotions and trauma of getting pregnant from rape was traumatic. I am 16 years old and still attending school. I'm trying to complete my school year so I can move on to Unitec to get a diploma in veterinary nursing.

My baby girl, Payton Dakota Jones, was taken from me when I was only 21 weeks pregnant. Payton had Turner's syndrome. She also had hydrops and a cystic hygroma on the back of her neck and head causing her whole body to swell up with fluid. My journey was a long process, helped by my faith in God.

Up until I was 12 weeks pregnant I had no idea my baby was sick. At my 12-week scan they measured the space between the baby's neck and my womb. This space showed that Payton had a cystic hygroma on the back of her neck. At the time of my scan they didn't tell me anything, they just said congratulations on your pregnancy and have a nice day.

That night my midwife phoned to give me the bad news. When she told me I couldn't help but break into tears in front of my family – I couldn't speak. They all just sat in silence waiting to hear what was going on. I handed the phone to my mum. My mum cried after she hung up. I didn't want to tell anyone so my mum did. I cried so much that night that my mum and dad didn't know what to do, so they went and picked up one of my best friends, Heleni. She comforted me for ages, just talking to me and saying that the baby will make it and that God will heal her.

Throughout my pregnancy I kept being told by the doctors and mid-wives to terminate the baby, even when I was 18 weeks pregnant. They thought that it would be easier for me to kill my baby than to give her a chance to survive and just hope for the best. While I was pregnant I learnt not to listen to the specialists and midwives. If I had listened to them I wouldn't have gotten so far in my pregnancy and I wouldn't have felt that I'd done everything I could to help Payton.

I kept praying and hoping that one day one of my scans would show that nothing was wrong with her. But they never did. Instead she got worse and worse until the fluid was in her lungs and around her neck and hands. Even then I never gave up on her. My mum was with me for everything I went through. I also had Payton's godmother with me a lot of the time as well. Her name is Lineti. She was someone that I could always talk to and she organised our church to pray for Payton and me.

On 7 July I went for my 21-week scan. I was prepared like any other mum to see my baby's little heartbeat, and legs and arms waving and kicking around. Instead as the cold goo went on my belly everyone was in silence. I already knew from the minute she put the scanner on my belly that Payton Dakota Jones had passed away. Instead, the person scanning me kept dragging the scan on, waiting for a heartbeat, giving me false hope. I wanted to scream but instead silent tears rolled down my face as she told me that my daughter had passed away.

My mum and Payton's godmother Lineti were with me, comforting me in any way they could. They put us in a tiny room with four chairs and left us there for about half an hour to talk about what had just happened. I couldn't stop crying, we were all so confused. Soon after my scan the midwife came to talk to us about what was going to happen next. She gave me three pills to swallow to stop the hormones going to Payton and preparing my body for labour.

The pastors of my church came to my house to pray for Payton and me. They prayed for a miracle and told me that it wasn't over yet. Three days later I had to go back to the hospital to be induced. I was happy and excited because I thought God was going to work a miracle and save my baby girl.

Before they induced me I demanded another scan to double-check. Still no heartbeat, but I was still in denial thinking that she was going to come out crying and screaming like a live baby.

On 9 July, at 4.55pm, Payton Dakota Jones was born. I was in labour for five to six hours. She weighed 705 grams and she was 26cm long. She had everything: fingernails, hair, eyebrows, eyes (not open), lips and a cute little nose, even hands and feet. She was a fully formed baby. Holding onto her was really hard because she was so still. Her body was cold and so lifeless. I didn't even get to see the colour of her eyes or hear her cry. Nothing but her body lay in my arms. Still in denial that she had passed away, I waited patiently for her to cry.

It wasn't until the next day that I broke into tears uncontrollably. Lineti was with me at the time rubbing my back comforting me while I cried so loudly. My mum went down to get something to eat. They slept in the double bed beside mine, comforting me in my time of need. So many visitors came to see me and Payton while I was at the hospital and at home. I had three days to spend time with my baby girl at home before the funeral. Payton was never left alone. If I wasn't in the room someone else was there to hold her in her little basket that she was nicely resting in.

She was dressed in a white dress with her pink hat and pink blanket that I bought for her.

On Monday 12 July Payton Dakota Jones was buried at the cemetery. So many of my friends and family showed up to her funeral. The word had spread around my school and Heleni got a dance group to come – there were 60 girls in it! I was in that same group at the beginning of the year while I was pregnant.

My pastor took the ceremony and I wrote a speech that I read out before they buried her. Lineti's family sang four songs at the funeral, which was a really beautiful send-off for Payton. One of my friends, Louise, had brought a fake flower and everyone put one earring each on one of the petals to go on Payton's grave. Saying goodbye to my baby girl was so hard when all this time I'd prepared myself for having a little girl. I had to cancel lay-bys for things that I bought for her. I put all the clothes that my friends brought for her in a memory box.

I go down to the cemetery every day to spend time with Payton, whether it's raining or sunny. There has not been one day when she has not been brought up in a conversation or thought about. This little girl impacted on so many people's lives. Her life was not in vain. She has brought me closer to my family and friends, and I never regret going as far as I did in my pregnancy.

My older sister is also pregnant. She was only three weeks behind me, which makes it a lot more difficult to see her pregnancy going to plan, with me losing my baby. Losing my little girl was the worst thing I have ever had to go through, and I know that I will never be the same again.

Payton Dakota Jones will forever be in my heart and will always be recognised as my firstborn.

Most of mine are not in this world

Dave Trumm

30 October 2009

Dearest Peach,

It's your first birthday today. You have been crawling all over the place for a while now, even standing and trying a few tentative steps. The candle in the cake intrigues you but your brother has to blow it out since you can't quite manage that yet. But no, that's not how it turned out. You are only with us in spirit.

We miss you dear Peach. My life has changed so much since we lost you. I feel at times that there is a hole in my soul that can never be mended.

I read a book to your brother the other day. 'The Tear Thief'. In the book, a young spirit girl travels the world at night, visiting children who are crying. She gently takes the tears that fall down their cheeks, collects them in a bag, and then flies up to the moon and pours the tears into the moon. The moon shines with all the tears that she collected each night. Tears of grieving from loss are the brightest of all.

Are you our tear thief? Have you been taking my tears away and making the moon even brighter? Have you been taking the tears that your mother so quietly sheds and pouring them into the moon? When I see the moon shining so brightly, I especially think of you.

This is your day, my little angel. Your candle is burning.

Daddy loves you

My wife and I were very happy with our dear son, two years old at the time. We were pregnant again, planning to complete our family and to give our child a sibling. At 11 weeks in, we went to the hospital for a visit with the doctors since my wife had pre-eclampsia the first time around and they wanted to keep a close eye on her this time. Well, at the visit they decided to do a quick scan.

Right away, we could see there was no heartbeat! The shock was intense. My mind was racing. What was going on? How could this be? What happened? What does this mean? We have lost our baby! We cried and cried. It hit me so hard. Up until then I was blissfully unaware of the other side of pregnancy – baby loss – and just what it means.

To have the baby just taken away from us like that was not fair! All those hopes and plans we had for our baby girl were gone, just like that. My dear wife was leaving the country on a work-related trip only one week after we found we had lost our baby, so she went in for a D&C (dilatation and curettage). When I asked her how she felt in the recovery room after the operation, she said *"not pregnant"* and cried and cried. It tore me up inside.

Early on, I discovered an online forum and also relied on friends in my Plunket group for support. One of them accompanied me to the hospital to pick up our baby after the D&C. She was a true angel. I felt like I needed to express my feelings about the loss and find every way I could to help validate just how much it had affected me, like naming our baby, burying our baby, talking with others, and writing. I was emotionally fragile. It was the most I had ever cried in my life.

The words of an older manager at work came back to haunt me. About three years earlier, when we were pregnant with our son, he told me that their little girl was the best thing that had ever happened in their lives. The most joy they have ever felt. Then they tried for a second one and failed. He said it was the saddest time in their lives. They went from the very top of happiness to the very bottom of sadness.

For me, nights were the worst. I typically remember my dreams, but now I wish that I didn't. Before picking up our baby I would dream that I was picking up a full-sized baby girl. I had many dreams about raising a second child, only to wake up with reality crashing back in. Others were about never conceiving again or having multiple miscarriages. I found I did not want to go to sleep for fear of what dreams lay ahead.

We buried our baby girl, planted a peach tree and pink daffodils, and named our baby Peach. Our son knows the area as somewhere significant to us. He often said out of the blue *"I want to go see Peach and say hi"*, which brought tears to my eyes. So I would put him in his little red wagon and pull him to the sunny part of the yard where she is buried. He would climb out, walk over to her, wave and say *"hi Peach"*.

Four months after we lost Peach we lost our next baby, Cherry. Morning sickness had suspiciously subsided so we had an early scan at nine weeks. I felt the same amount of intense grief and sadness but much less shock. The innocence of pregnancy had been lost. Following a natural miscarriage, we buried Cherry next to her sister and planted a cherry tree.

Fertility clinic testing showed that there was no reason for our miscarriages except that age was against us. A third try resulted in a third miscarriage nearly a year after Cherry was buried. BB was buried next to her sisters. At this point we called it quits and began to attend the yearly Sands Christmas candle lighting service and the Baby Loss Awareness Week service.

And I continued to write letters to my lost children.

Dear Angel Baby, precious one,

Your spirit and soul have only just left us, your body still being carried by your mother. You were to be our miracle baby, our Christmas baby, with a 31 December due date, and our third and last try at having a sibling for your brother.

Your final resting place awaits you. It is next to your two sisters. I pray that you choose to let go, to depart from your mother so that we can finally put you to rest and relieve your mother of ongoing morning sickness.

Someday I will explain to your brother how hard we tried to have another sibling for him. And that he does have three other siblings, it's just that they are not here with us. He will then remember that special place in the yard, that place where we often visit and he waves hello to Peach and to Cherry and now, soon, to you too.

I grieve for you, and for the life here that could have been. I grieve again for your dearest mother and the intense emotional pain that she is, once again, going through. I grieve for my dear son. His fate to be an only child has now been sealed. And I grieve for myself, for I feel as though, with your loss, I have suffered more this past year than any time before.

Please, be free wherever you are. We can only hope that you are in a better place than here. We will never forget you, our miracle baby, our Christmas baby.

Daddy loves you

It has now been 18 months since our last and final miscarriage. The grief and sadness I feel from our losses is fading but at times can be quite raw. There are reminders, which can bring me back to the grief of those early days: pregnant women, families with two or more children, pregnancy stories on TV or in the paper, announcements of pregnancies, the list goes on.

As a man, I have felt very alone over these last few years. Men are expected to be stoic, to try to fix problems (like one can fix the grief from miscarriage!) and to shrug our shoulders and move on. Aren't they?

I found I could not do any of these. I felt like I had failed. Although reception on the online forum has been outstanding, I have often felt odd about the intensity with which the miscarriages have hit me, considering that all the other members of the forum are women. I can only conclude that I am not alone, and that most other men choose to grieve for their loss more privately.

I've reached a point in my life where I am ready to raise a family. Most life goals have been met, I'm satisfied with my career achievements, and I'm ready to show my children the wonders of the world. It's just that most of my children are not in this world.

The hurt of those days after

Anonymous

We started trying for a baby in November 2004, and yes we remember the month because every year is an anniversary of something we don't want to celebrate; the fact that we don't have the baby we so long for.

Because we were what is classed as young when we started trying (23 and 24) we had heard that you should try for a year before seeing a doctor; so we did that and at the end of that year of trying we weren't pregnant. That year was so difficult because we were sure we would get pregnant – well of course we thought that, why wouldn't we?

We went to our GP and had some tests done, which indicated that my husband had a low count and issues with morphology. We were referred to a fertility specialist and had more thorough tests done, which indicated that hubby's sperm count was borderline as was his morphology, and that I may not ovulate every month. We were told that if we were with different partners we could probably get pregnant; that was one of the most useful things anyone has ever said to us … NOT!

We were given our options and started on clomiphene. The specialist told us that he was pretty confident we would be pregnant with the help of it. Well – at the end of six cycles we weren't. We were given our next option which was IVF (in vitro fertilisation). After some discussion we decided we would do it, as it would all be worth it if we ended up with a baby in our arms.

I don't think anything can prepare you or your body for the physical and mental challenges that IVF brings. The injections every day is the easy part; it's the waiting for results, waiting to hear if your levels are right, waiting to hear how many embryos have fertilised, waiting, waiting, waiting. Our life revolved around blood tests, scans (to check my uterus lining), injection training, meetings with nurses and specialists. It definitely is not the 'have sex at the right time of the month and get pregnant' scenario you think of when first deciding to have a baby.

I describe my journey with IVF as a roller coaster. There's the ups – at the beginning there is so much hope that this is going to work – and then at the end the downs when you find out it hasn't worked, and then all the ups and downs in between.

Then there is the waiting for two weeks before the blood test – what is usually referred to in 'IVF circles' as the dreaded two-week wait. You know you have the embryo on board in the beginning, but towards the end of the two-week wait you don't know if it has resulted in you being pregnant. Then there is the waiting for 'the phone call' after the morning blood test to see if it was all worth it; in the end, for us, both of our IVF cycles resulted in the nurse phoning to say *"I am sorry, the test is negative"*. In both cycles I had bleeding before the test but I was still secretly hoping that it was implantation bleeding or some other bleeding but it wasn't.

How do I describe the hurt of those days after the negative results? I think it would have been less painful to have just taken my heart out altogether? And who is there to talk to who understands? Where is the person who has walked in your shoes?

Being 'infertile' is so isolating. I can't thank my family enough for their support, although it was from the other side of the world in England where they live; the daily phone calls from my mum helped even if I was just sitting on the phone sobbing. I never will forget the feeling; the broken feeling of finding out we weren't successful in achieving our dream.

There are very few people in my life who know about our situation, and that is by choice because I don't want to feel judged. I feel enough like a failure as a woman, and as a wife, let alone dealing with judgement or pity from others. I also haven't told many people because my intention in telling people is to have support or some compassion; however, we have not received it. So after some bad experiences, sometimes resulting in the closing of doors on friendships, we decided this is something we will keep pretty much to ourselves.

Then there are the unhelpful words of people who truly don't under-stand, like *"it's okay, just relax and it will happen"* or *"go on holiday it will happen"*.

Please, if you don't have any really helpful advice, don't open your mouth.

It's funny (well, not funny ha ha), but I had a family member say to me the other day *"when are you going to have kids? You better hurry up, you're running out of time"*.

For the record I have only just turned 30, and secondly I know I am getting older in reproductive terms, but comments like that are not helpful, even if you are not struggling to conceive!

Now, sitting at the end of our journey, I feel like I am a different person in some ways. I find it so difficult to pretend to be happy for people in my life who announce they are pregnant; well, I don't know if that's the 'politically correct' thing to say, but in my heart it's the truth – the hurt is so immense. I told my mum once that this pain is on par with the pain of suddenly losing my dad when I was a teenager; a different pain but on the same level.

Like other situations where grief is involved I am managing to live my day-to-day life and am generally happy. We recently celebrated our four-year wedding anniversary, which was an anniversary I did want to celebrate. I have the most amazing, wonderful husband and am so grateful to whomever sent him to me; one thing I know is that whether we have a baby or not we will always have each other, and how can I not be happy with that.

There are times that remind me of our 'situation' that sometimes pop up, be it after seeing those gorgeous giggling baby ads on TV or having a work colleague announce she is pregnant when they weren't even trying.

People may say they understand, but how can they if they haven't been through it? How can they understand the longing of wanting to be a mother and not knowing if it is ever going to happen?

Lastly, where to for us now? Well, we can't afford private IVF treatment. We would go through it all in a heartbeat if we could, but we can't. It hurts so bad to know that possibly money is the only barrier between us and our baby. Others may say that they would do anything to have a baby, but if you don't have the money you can't make it appear from nowhere. The government only pay for two publicly funded IVF treatments.

We have talked about adoption on and off, but we both feel that adoption isn't right for us and at the end of the day what's right for us and our situation is what matters. There are many who go from unsuccessful IVF cycles to the adoption pool. It is great that that option is there, it's just not for us.

So really, where to from here? Well, the answer's nowhere. The specialist has told us he can't see why we can't get pregnant naturally and that it might happen or it might not. So more waiting I guess, but along with that wait we move on with the rest of our lives. I can't lie, but every month if my period is a couple of days late I hope that a miracle has happened to us.

One more try

Jodi Oldham

I have always loved looking after children. First I became a teacher, then couldn't wait to be a mother. My husband and I used to joke about having a big family. At our wedding, people even made bets that I'd be pregnant within a year, despite our OE travel plans!

When we did start trying for a baby, it just didn't happen. Friends around us seemed to be falling pregnant instantly, but not us.

I would get my hopes up each month, with lots of phantom pregnancy symptoms, only to be disappointed time and time again. All the clichéd advice came out – *"you're working too hard, go on holiday"*, *"it will happen when you stop thinking about it"*. But after nearly two years of this emotional roller coaster we decided to try IVF (in vitro fertilisation).

I used to be scared of needles, but had to get over that quickly! My husband had the lovely task of injecting me every day, then there were lots of blood tests and scans. Getting my eggs out was so painful I kicked the doctor in the head. Two little embryos were put back, we waited anxiously, then finally got the great news! We were pregnant!

I had the most wonderful pregnancy. I revelled in all the pregnancy symptoms and was even delighted to throw up! Just one of the embryos had taken, which doctors were pleased about – less risk.

It was great to get past the 12-week point, then my baby starting kicking early and growing quickly. All the scans, nuchal fold tests and blood tests indicated a 'bonny healthy baby'. Finally we could decorate the nursery and buy baby clothes. We were really looking forward to meeting our little one.

But as I reached the third trimester, my baby was gradually kicking less. Everyone reassured me, saying babies don't have as much room to move now. Even the specialist said the chance of losing a baby at 30 weeks was only one in 2,000. I tried so hard not to worry.

My last antenatal appointment, at 32 weeks, was on a beautiful sunny day in June. I was concerned that the movements had changed, and was looking forward to more reassurance. I had thought about looking around the maternity unit afterwards or maybe going for a walk in the park. What happened instead was just so awful. The movements weren't movements at all but Braxton Hicks contractions. I'll never forget the radiographer's cold hard words – *"well, the baby has died"*. Our darling, precious, long-awaited baby. Part of me died too.

Ringing my husband was heartbreaking – he was so looking forward to having this baby. The following day I gave birth to a gorgeous little boy who looked like his daddy. We called him William – a family name on both sides.

The next few days were surreal – leaving hospital, arranging the funeral, flowers and cards arriving at the door. Our friends and family were very upset and at first we were actually comforting them. I think I was focusing on the birth of my baby rather than his death. I kept waking up during the night remembering my little boy's face and being overwhelmed with love for him.

The loss didn't really sink in until after William's funeral. Then reality hit hard – his poor little life was over before it had even begun. And ours had been ripped apart. I was angry and scared of everything – losing my husband, driving my car, going back to work, etc. I didn't feel whole – it was like my arm or leg had been cut off. I kept thinking why us, why our little boy, why, why, why? Did I work too hard, eat something I shouldn't have, roll over in bed the wrong way? But I had been so careful! The questions and the tears were constant.

Finally we got the autopsy results – our little boy had Down syndrome. That only made me love him more, but it did stop some of the questions.

Gradually I started rebuilding my life. Talking to people from Sands was very helpful. Exercise became a daily ritual, first walking, then swimming and later aerobics. Career decisions were hard, all I really wanted to be was William's mum. But I missed being around children and eventually went back to my teaching job.

The staff were supportive and the children (five to six years) were great. Their honesty was so refreshing. They just wanted to know, did I have a boy or a girl and what did I call him? Very important questions that most adults don't ask, they can't get past the word 'stillborn'. Our wonderful nieces and nephews talked openly about their baby cousin in heaven.

We had good support from family and close friends. They know how special William is and some of them grieved too. They kept saying *'it's so unfair'*. But life is unfair – you just have to take what happens and make the best of it.

After a few months, we decided to have another try at IVF. We were longing more than ever for a baby to have and to hold, to nurture, to watch grow. We had got so close! We knew we could never replace William. He will always be our firstborn, and our love for him will always be strong. I felt like he'd never left me – just moved from my tummy to my heart. But we had some little frozen embryos – maybe one would become his brother or sister.

We had six frozen embryos replaced, month after month, but none of them took. Live healthy babies were being born all around us. Some close relatives and friends had their babies within a few months of

William's birth. It was a constant reminder of what should have been. Visiting new babies was difficult as were children's birthday parties. Christenings were especially painful. We avoided these as much as possible. Jealousy was a horrible feeling that churned me up inside. I tried to be happy for others but was terribly sad for us.

We started another full round of IVF the year after and … I got pregnant again! We were delighted, but very anxious. I had some bleeding at seven weeks, which was terrifying – we rushed in for a scan, only to be reassured that all was well, with not just one but two babies. Twins! We had always wanted twins! Our spirits lifted and we shared the news with our families. People started getting excited. Good things do happen to those who wait!

We lost them both, one after the other, within a few weeks. Their little heartbeats just failed to show up on the scans. I really hate scans now! It was put down to sheer bad luck, and we were advised to try again. And we were still determined! We had a few frozen embryos replaced but again none of them took.

The following year we went for our third IVF cycle and I was pregnant again – for four days. The first blood test was positive, the second negative. This is what's called a biochemical pregnancy. More bad luck. Why did this keep happening to us?

It was now nearly two years since William's birth (and death). I still thought about him all the time, and the other tiny babies we lost but never really knew.

I was starting to face the possibility that I may not ever give birth to a live baby. This was devastating. It still felt like my whole purpose in life was to be a mother. I treasured the memories of that wonderful pregnancy with

William and thought *"at least I had that"*. I tried to stay positive and made lists of all the other good things that happened in my life.

We got a lovely little dog, who wasn't a baby substitute but did make us feel like a family. We'd always wanted a dog – we just thought we'd have children first. But life wasn't turning out the way we'd planned.

We wondered where to go from here. I couldn't imagine life without children and kept thinking *"don't give up, don't ever give up"*. But IVF treatment is so stressful and expensive. Where do you draw the line? When do you say enough is enough? Maybe it was time to look at other options. However, we decided to give IVF one more try …

Eight months later, I gave birth to beautiful, healthy twin girls. Two little miracles! We look at these delightful children and still can't believe they are really ours. Such a long journey, but so worth it in the end. We are very proud, very grateful parents.

I just didn't want to let him go

Monique Jonasen

Sunday 5 January 2003 we went to hospital as I had a show of blood in the morning, only to realise that I was in labour. I was rushed down to hospital. I was only 26 weeks pregnant.

On Wednesday 8 January 2003 Brodie was born weighing 996 grams. He was one of the biggest in his room with other premmies around the same age. It was one of the most exciting, yet scary, days of our lives.

Everything was going so well, he was doing what he was meant to and he was so perfect, nothing was wrong. Day 11 was upon us and I had to shoot home to see my specialist. I didn't want to leave my boy.

I was getting ready to leave home to drive back down to the hospital that morning. At 7am the phone rang, and the doctor said *"Monique, Brodie's had a rough night, how long until you can get here?"* I said *"three hours at the quickest, I'll leave now."*

Not even ten minutes later the phone rang again. *"Monique, I'm sorry, Brodie has passed away."*

All I remember doing is screaming and dropping to the floor. My dad took the phone and spoke to the doctor, and arranged for us to get down there as soon as possible.

I was in no state to ring my husband and tell him. My father took care of it. It seemed like so long until my husband got home, and the drive to the hospital took forever.

Walking back into SCBU (Special Case Baby Unit) was horrible. We were escorted into a tiny room, and there on the bed lay my tiny baby dressed and placed in a tiny cane basket. He was cold and stiff, and still had blood coming out of his nose. I will never forget that moment, it was horrible. I just couldn't stop screaming and crying.

After a short time the doctor came in and explained to us that he had had a lung haemorrhage and they couldn't keep him alive, so he drowned in his own blood. They said they were glad that I wasn't there to see it as it was not nice.

After many hours had passed we had to hand Brodie back so they could do an autopsy and embalm him, before being flown back to Napier airport for our funeral director to pick him up.

When we saw him at the funeral home he looked like an old man, he was so wrinkly, it was horrible. We had a beautiful white satin-lined coffin and we dressed him in a white gown. We put a bonnet on his head, and as we moved him we saw that there was blood at the back of his head and on the satin. They had opened up his head in the autopsy. I was so angry. How could they do that? It felt as though he had been treated with little respect. I didn't even want the autopsy done, but the law can override parents' wishes anyway.

Brodie's funeral came around – 10am. This was the hardest day I have ever been through. There were over 100 people. We had a song, *Angels*, by John Farnham. I just didn't want to let him go. This was a son that I had longed for and now he was being taken away from me. *"Why, why!"* I just wanted it to be a bad dream and go away.

Dealing with the grief after the funeral was really hard. I felt anger, sadness, and hatred.

People said things like *"Oh, it was meant to be"* or *"Never mind love, you'll have more"* or *"you'll be pregnant again before you know it!"*

This went on for ages. I was ready to hit some people.

For a long time afterwards I struggled to deal with everyday life. Seeing pregnant women and newborn babies was really hard. Hearing that someone we knew was pregnant or hearing about someone that didn't deserve a child was exceptionally hard.

We tried to get on with life, as difficult as it was. We tried for another baby about seven months later. It took five years to have another baby.

Kade was born at 29 weeks. I was a mess when he was born as I thought we were going to lose him too. We didn't and he is a happy, healthy two-year-old now.

Kade knows he has a big brother called Brodie. He says *"hello Brodie"* every time we go past the cemetery and toot. He also sees a star in the sky and points to it and says *"Brodie"* – we nicknamed Brodie 'brodstar' as he was a little miracle in our lives.

Although this horrible experience happened nearly eight years ago, we still have bad days, we still cry, and it still feels as though it was only yesterday. If anything, it has made us stronger as a couple and more demanding and forthright in fighting for our son Kade's welfare.

If you can get through the loss of a child together you can get through anything!

A greater knowing of what I have lost

Nicky

Here are some of my thoughts from the first few days after my second miscarriage. They certainly illustrate how the whole process made me feel.

21 September 2009

I'm having a scan tomorrow that will probably show me my baby has died. I've been living in limbo for four weeks. I had pain at $4\frac{1}{2}$ weeks … the doctor thought I had a possible ectopic pregnancy. So I had a scan at five weeks and five days. The scan showed an empty sac measuring five weeks. No heartbeat, perhaps too early to tell?

Hormone levels were very good throughout. Fourteen days later I had a second scan that showed the baby was six weeks and two days, no heartbeat. The baby had grown from the first scan but should have been measuring seven weeks. So I went home to miscarry.

Eleven days later nothing has happened. A week ago I had a very good blood test that showed an HCG (human chorionic gonadotrophin) increase of 50,000 over four days – I was also feeling very symptomatic. So the doctor thought it was possibly a good sign. Perhaps my dates were just out.

Last Friday I realised I wasn't feeling sick. Bloods showed a 50,000 decline in HCG (only four days from the previous high result). I should be nine weeks and three days tomorrow.

Don't know whether to ask for a D&C (dilatation and curettage) or just keep waiting. It's horrible just waiting and waiting and nothing happens.

I am thinking it may be best to finish this. But reading some of the D&C posts (online forum) has been horrific!

I live in a rural community and I have to travel an hour and a half to the nearest hospital. The hospital is staffed by locums so I am hoping there is a specialist on duty tomorrow. The nurse at the medical centre here said there were no guarantees I could have a D&C straight away due to that factor. I may have to wait until my doctor is available. I hope they are as I'm ready to move on now.

The alternative is to drive to the next big hospital, an additional three hours away.

24 September 2009

I've just read what I have written and I sound like I am an emotional hormonal, crazy mum … oh well here goes …

On Tuesday my pregnancy was officially nine weeks and two days. We drove to the hospital for the scan. For some strange reason I was very clinical when I got there. I wasn't emotional at all when I actually had the scan at 10.20am. I told the scanner operator that this scan was not going to produce good news so let's see what's been going on.

The baby was difficult to find and had not changed in size since the previous scan. But the foetal sac had grown HUGE – way too huge (I had thought I was starting to show at eight weeks and now I know why). That is why my HCG levels had been going up so much. The sac appeared to be acting on its own, doing a good job of growing. A blood test on Tuesday revealed that, yes, the HCG levels were definitely on the way down.

Because I had been in limbo for two weeks I was able to ask for the D&C. I had the pill that softens the cervix first, to help bring things along.

When I got to theatre at 3.15pm I lost the plot and bawled and bawled. It was at the final realisation that this pregnancy was really truly over. All my hopes and dreams for him or her gone.

I woke up from theatre at 4.10pm still bawling … so much so that I wonder if I bawled when I was out to it.

The staff were fantastic and I stayed just one night because the bleeding was normal. The D&C itself went well. I have found it much easier than the previous natural miscarriage that I had. With that miscarriage I found it devastating every time I went to the toilet and found big clots.

My only regret this time is that nobody said anything to me about retaining the baby. I would have taken her or him home for a burial under a new tree or something.

I've been bawling ever since. I just can't stop. It hasn't been 48 hours yet, so I suppose I'm allowed to. Sitting here in my PJs now, the kids have to be at school in 20 minutes … don't know if they'll get there!

I'm having cramps again this morning front and back – I didn't have any at all yesterday so I hope I'm normal. Perhaps it's just my uterus going back to normal size.

I had kept my original pregnancy test but it isn't where I thought I had safely left it. So that sent me bawling because now I have no physical evidence at home of the pregnancy ever existing. All I have for the memory box is my hospital band and a cake of soap from the hospital. Suppose that's better than nothing.

My two kids, aged five and six, know nothing of what's going on, apart from I went to hospital for a night. I've managed not to bawl in front of them so far. I don't know if it's a good idea to tell them because they didn't know I was pregnant.

My six-year-old would probably understand but then she might tell people.

I'm struggling with feelings of anger towards my husband. I've read that could happen because men deal with this differently from us … but … he just has no emotion at all about any of it. He told me he doesn't feel anything. I said to him *"well can't you feel some empathy for me then, if not for yourself"*?

There's NO compassion from him and it's really peeing me off. He's clinical and says nothing at all if I tell him anything of my feelings … nothing. I have had to ask for hugs as he isn't forth coming … he hasn't told me he loves me or anything … he's just keeping his distance.

I told him this morning I'm trying to make a memory box and he didn't even comment. I gave him a miscarriage pamphlet from the hospital so he could read about how my feelings would be, and it hasn't changed anything about his reaction to me. Perhaps I should write him a note telling him all I need is to be shown some love from him.

Other husbands behave better than this surely? I feel this could actually be the end of us. How can a man who is supposed to love me be so distant at a time like this? I feel completely alone in all of this … he hasn't lost anything as far as he's concerned.

I've already had horrible reactions from some people. Not many family members knew I was pregnant. My sister did. On Monday, the day before I had the scan and D&C, she said to me *"well you have to put this in perspective, I've got a friend who had breast cancer with three young kids and that was just devastating. You've got two healthy kids anyway. Be thankful for that"*.

Yes I know that! Yes cancer is waaaaaaaaaaaaay more devastating and on the meter of bad things in life that would be far worse. So is the fact my friend had stillborn twins, another had a cot death. YES all far worse. Yes I do have two kids so I am lucky … that in itself gives me a greater knowing of what I have lost.

But surely I'm allowed a few days to cry and feel sad and grieve for this immense loss from my life. I had already imagined holding that wee newborn for the first time. The sleepy cuddles you get only when they are very new. The smell of them, the feel of them … everything about that baby I had imagined. I had imagined the first fluttering kicks in my tummy. The big kicks later on … the big swelling belly that gets in the way of everything and makes your feet disappear. I had even imagined as far as age five when he/she went to school. I've known all of that and I was looking forward to it again. I think that is the true nature of the loss that you feel.

It's like you don't want to go through a miscarriage without anyone knowing. You want acknowledgement of the child's existence. But if you tell some people you get shot down.

In my heart I know my baby is in peace and in a good place.

Well, enough said … got it all out though!

24 September 2009

When I was home alone this morning I was a mess. A friend came around and 'rescued' me from my despair. The kids are home now and my son has a friend around to keep him occupied. I've been carrying on with normal tasks but my tummy is very crampy so I've got the 'can't-be-bothered' thing going on right now.

I realise how lucky I have been to have produced two healthy children. I met a lady on Monday who had 12 first trimester miscarriages and a stillborn at 24 weeks. Finally at the age of 42 she had IVF (in vitro fertilisation) using donated eggs and produced two beautiful twin girls who are the absolute love of her life.

I know I'll get through this as I did before … last time I clung onto the fact that I would try again and get that baby back. Which I did! I'm not sure about that this time … I really did want another child but at this exact moment I don't know if I can risk having this happen again.

Miscarriage is so silent. We act very Victorian about it, all quiet and behind closed doors. Both my kids got up for news at school yesterday and told their respective classes *"my mum's in hospital and she's sick"*, so today at school their teachers and half the parents were asking what was wrong. I didn't know what to say … *"I had some tests done and had to have a small operation but I'm fine now"*.

Why didn't I just say … *"I had a miscarriage and had a D&C"* … but you don't do you, it's not the done thing … then people wouldn't know what to say to you.

My GP rang today to see how I was. He assured me my age wouldn't have affected my fertility (I'm 36). He assured me my chances of miscarrying again are only the same as a first-time pregnancy. He assured me the stress I was under during the pregnancy wouldn't have caused it … more likely it was a 'normal' genetic problem and it was nature's way of taking care of it. Who knows?

I'm planning a weekend away in Christchurch this weekend with the kids, bad weather forecast and all. I need retail therapy and can't face being stuck indoors all weekend home alone (husband has trip pre-planned). I'd rather be in a big city just in case any infection occurs post-op. I live in the wop-wops so it will feel safer to be in a city.

I'm going to find a tree to plant and buy something for the memory box.

24 September 2009

Hubby came home in a better mood. Someone at work asked him why he'd been off work and he blurted out the real answer. His work is very blokey so I think the other guy took off. He didn't know what to say! He told his pay-lady too and she put his leave down as sick leave. Given he told me that, it makes me realise that he is thinking about things – even if he's useless with the actual event.

My boss at work knows why I'm off work and she has been fantastic! She's great with people and not just a boss but kind of like a life coach too. She's very spiritual and has been able to offer me real comfort with thinking of the baby in the afterlife and has suggested some good ideas on ways to remember and acknowledge the baby. And ways to keep my mind busy so I don't blubber all day.

I'm not looking forward to next week when I'm back at work and people start asking why I was away.

I live in a small town and moved here 12 months ago. I don't have many friends here but there are a couple of good ones who have had miscarriages themselves. One friend spent most of the day with me because I asked her to. I don't seem to be good in the mornings so I'll have to keep myself busy. I think I need some real sleep too, that will help!

30 September 2009

Had the histology report back and they found nothing wrong. So was it stress? Was it due to the virus I had at the five to six week mark? Was it just not meant to be? Who knows?

I also had the scan reports back and that confirmed the baby sac continued to grow for a further three weeks after the baby had died. Apparently that's not very common.

13 October 2009

Three weeks since I had the D&C, and I am feeling a little better. I had heaps of energy at the weekend for the first time in about two months. I finally stopped bleeding on Sunday (fingers crossed). Week two after the D&C I had an infection, and once that was over I started to come right.

I haven't been bawling as much, but today I can't seem to stop. I think it has something to do with watching the news. That poor little girl in Auckland.

I feel so sad and I think my emotions are still quite raw so I am susceptible to a good old bawling session. Everything sets me off.

Then I watched *Good Morning* with the article on Baby Loss Awareness Week, that set me off again.

I don't have anyone to talk to about my feelings. I think the couple of friends who I could talk to are sick of me talking about it. They redirect me and tell me about worse situations that are really terrible. I think they think I should be over it by now.

I definitely coped better with the first miscarriage that I had years ago. I didn't have anyone to talk to much then either, but I had a nine-month-old at the time and I was too busy to stop and think about it. Plus I was able to try again straight away.

A year on … October 2010

After this miscarriage I couldn't let the pregnancy go.

I spent the next seven months living a virtual pregnancy. *"I should be seven months now"* etc. I didn't start to feel 'normal' until the estimated due date had past.

I felt I couldn't talk about it out loud to anyone. People didn't want to hear about the grief I had for a baby that was just a 'product of conception'.

I often felt jealous of people having babies. I lost a lot of joy in the world. I just never felt happy. In May this year, a month after the due date, I confessed to a group of friends how grieved I had been. They had no idea as I shut it all away.

Recently I have made a concerted effort to let it go. I am feeling happier and accepting of what happened.

I really want to be pregnant again. But I'm having fertility issues. Bit sad about that. I am about to embark on some fertility testing.

I'm 37 and have been trying for a third child for almost two years. I am very thankful for the two kids I do have.

Twin to twin

Tiffiny

If getting pregnant after only one attempt wasn't surprising enough, at our 12-week scan we were completely blown away when the sonographer asked *"how do you feel about two?"* I was pregnant with twins.

Like most people I confidently and excitedly stated to anyone who would listen that I was 'having twins'. We shopped for two of everything and I expanded at an amazing rate (at five months I was already the size of a 36-week pregnancy). I was constantly tired and was becoming uncomfortable quite quickly, but the joy of thinking that I had two wee babies inside cheered me up when I was cross and grumpy.

I was still in a haze of exhaustion and happiness at a 17-week scan on a Friday morning to confirm how many placentas and amniotic sacs there were, and the size of the babies. Each baby had its own sac attached to one placenta – identical twins. I was too excited seeing them waving and kicking each other on screen to notice the sonographer looking increasingly worried, but my partner Max was paying more attention and he left feeling slightly nervous. At 3pm that afternoon our doctor rang me at work. *"I want you to go home. We think there's something wrong with the babies."*

I felt like I was going to be sick. The doctor briefly mentioned Twin to Twin Transfusion Syndrome (TTTS) and the fact that one baby wasn't growing as well as the other. I was to be urgently referred to the High Risk Clinic at the hospital and spend the weekend resting.

Once home, I immediately looked up TTTS on the internet. Due to irregular connections to the placenta, one twin was receiving more blood etc than the other. This twin has to do more work pumping blood and is often larger and is known as the donor twin (polyhydramnious), while the other is starved for nutrient and is known as the recipient, or stuck, twin (oligohydramnious).

The statistics were horrible – only 20% of TTTS pregnancies ended with a live baby, with surviving twins at an increased chance of heart, lung, kidney and liver problems, and a much greater likelihood of complications such as cerebral palsy. By the time we saw the High Risk Team the following Tuesday we were both stressed, scared and confused.

I was told that I needed to keep the babies inside and healthy for as long as possible. We would aim for 32 weeks but could deliver at 26 – 28 weeks if absolutely necessary. I was told to take extended leave or quit my job as I would likely be on bed rest, in hospital, for two or three months.

The next five weeks held scans each week, and the twins, now called 'Poly' and 'Ollie' for their respective sizes, seemed to be doing well.

On Tuesday 12 February, at our weekly scan at nearly 23 weeks, things had abruptly worsened. My cervix size had changed and the doctor was worried. I was immediately admitted to hospital and scheduled for a second amnio reduction (a rather uncomfortable procedure where two large needles are inserted into Poly's amniotic sac and between one and two litres of liquid are slowly drawn off). This was to happen before a cervical cerclage operation was performed to sew me shut and keep the twins safe for a little longer.

After two days of nil by mouth the cerclage was performed, with the risk that it might stimulate labour instead of slowing it down. Within two hours the worst had happened – while the operation had gone well, contractions started shortly after.

The next two days were the worst in my life. For six hours I was given oral medication every 15 minutes to stop the contractions. When this failed I was put on the 'hard stuff' intravenously. Labour stopped around 10.30pm and Max went home, but I was kept in the delivery suite as this was the only place where I could be constantly monitored. With 13 holes, tubes and drips, a catheter, and people giving birth all around, I spent the night crying and telling my babies to hold on and stay inside a little bit longer.

At 8am the next morning a Doppler scan resulted in more bad news. Max was sent for urgently and we were asked to make a decision to terminate the pregnancy totally, selectively terminate the smaller twin in a risky operation that would have to be performed in America or England, or wait it out and risk them both. It is a decision no future parent should have to make, and by now I hated the words 'terminate' and 'viable'.

In the end, nature made the decision for us and I was in labour again within the hour. This time it couldn't be stopped.

We were made as comfortable as possible and, after a long day, a bed was brought in so Max could stay the night. My waters were broken the next morning and, after 23 hours and the enormous help of the midwife, a very tiny, beautiful baby was born – Georgia Beverly. We were warned that the babies might gasp for breath but, at a day under 23 weeks, they were too small to live, even with intervention. Georgia went one better and let out a cry to announce her arrival. She was handed to me, and although I desperately wanted to hold her, I still had work to do. She was handed to a father who was adamant that he did not want to touch either of the babies. With no other option, he held her in his arms and was not without one of the girls until we left the hospital.

Grace Ellen was born five minutes later and, despite being the smaller twin and in so much trouble internally, cried even louder than her sister. They weighed 500 and 400 grams respectively and both girls lived over an hour – just long enough to hold them and 'tell them that we loved them' as Max would later write. Then with the midwife's help we washed and dressed them, and took hand- and foot-prints and a roll of photos. These few things have become very precious.

It's almost nine years now since the girls were born and I've learnt that even such short lives can make a huge difference. Max and I were completely altered by the girls, and our lives have changed direction because of them. We are now about to celebrate another Christmas with our third and fourth children – the third was a healthy baby boy conceived five months to the day after his sisters died. He was a startlingly wonderful baby (born two days early on Easter Sunday – our 'new life' baby) and the sunny natures of him and his little brother make it easier to see in them all the things we lost with the girls, and still smile. Both subsequent pregnancies went well but I always said to people only that I was pregnant and never *"I'm having a baby"*, just in case.

The girls' deaths profoundly changed me, but their life has taught me some amazing lessons. Georgia and Grace were loved for the whole of their little lives and made a difference to many people. I am still proud to say that they are my children.

I carried on working as a midwife

Kerry Prendergast

I completed my midwifery training in 1977, the week that my daughter Melissa was born. I continued working at St Helens Hospital as a midwife. During this time I worked with many women who had suffered different kinds of birth tragedy, and I thought I was being really helpful but in hindsight I had no idea.

When Melissa was about 18 months old I got pregnant with my second child. I had severe morning sickness, much worse than the first time, and so I took medication to help. Near the end of my first trimester my GP told me to stop taking the medication immediately as new research had shown that it may cause birth defects. I stopped. For months I was anxious. What if something was wrong with the baby?

It was 1979 and I was under the care of a specialist. Scanning technology was very new at the time and he asked me if I was interested in participating in some scan research, which involved scanning me and my baby.

I got to 30 weeks and everything was going fine. However, the baby wasn't moving as much and I felt a bit uncomfortable. The scan had shown that the baby was a face presentation, which was very unusual, so the specialist sent me up for an X-ray. After the X-ray they asked me to wait, as they wanted to check some detail. Meanwhile they had phoned my husband to ask him to join me.

They had seen something abnormal. They thought that the baby had short arms and legs, a dwarf maybe, and it also had a big growth on the back of its head and multiple fractures. As a midwife, my immediate response was *"could it survive, what was wrong, what was the long-term prognosis?"* They simply didn't know.

It was traumatic walking round heavily pregnant and having well-meaning people saying *"you can't have long to go, you look great"*. I told many of them that things were not great, in fact my baby was probably going to die. I just couldn't cope with the remarks, so I stayed at home.

At 34 weeks I went into labour spontaneously. I was still working; I had to for my sanity. Everyone around me at work was devastated: the midwives, the doctors, the anaesthetists. I withdrew deeply into myself and was not able to respond emotionally to anyone.

The obstetrician wanted me to deliver the baby vaginally. I was terrified. In my mind I was going to be delivering a monster. I did not want this child to survive longer than necessary, and so didn't want any intervention to keep the baby alive.

Our baby boy lived for 40 minutes and had 88 fractures; every bone in his tiny body was broken. Some were broken in utero, others during the birth. His head looked funny because it was badly fractured. The pain of those breaks must have been terrible. He was wrapped and put in a cot to quietly die.

I held him very briefly, he had white hair and blue eyes. He wasn't a monster, he was beautiful. Unfortunately my only physical evidence of Paul is an early scan photo and a tombstone. And then I have my memories …

The hospital chaplain/priest baptised him in the theatre and named him Paul, the same name as my husband, but he didn't even ask us first, he just named him. My husband felt like part of him had died and that, consequently, he was burying himself.

The funeral home made a traumatic mistake. We wanted Paul to be buried in his own grave with his own headstone. They had buried him in a communal grave and he had to be exhumed.

Then a mistake took place at the specialist's rooms. I went back for my six-week postnatal check and the receptionist asked *"where is your baby? There is no point coming in for a six-week check if you don't have your baby"*. How utterly insensitive!

Being a midwife and having a huge amount of experience dealing with death and grief as a nurse did not prepare me for the pain of losing a child. It didn't help that for four weeks I knew he was likely to die. It did not lessen the intensity or the longevity of my grief.

After losing Paul I found it very traumatic seeing mothers and children. I could not stand hearing of cases where babies were unwanted or where there was violence. How could these people not appreciate the precious gift that they had been given!

Every Sunday we used to have lunch with my husband's parents and family. My sister-in-law had a baby shortly before we lost Paul. We immediately stopped seeing them, the pain was too intense for me. We would still go to the lunches but made sure we left before they arrived or we arrived after they had left. This lasted for a year and I felt so guilty about it, but I just could not bear to see or hold another baby, especially ones with any emotional attachment.

However, I carried on working as a midwife; I actually went back within a month, I had to. I rationalised that I had no emotional attachment to these women or their babies and so I was able to work. It seemed bizarre that I could cope with it but I could logically rationalise it as it was my job, but I could not cope with seeing the babies of friends and family. I had to work for sanity.

People could be extremely insensitive and would say *"it only lived for an hour"*. But I was not grieving for the 34 weeks that he was inside me and his short life, it was the lifetime of hopes and expectations that I held for him. He was going to be the most perfect baby, the one created in the fantasy of my mind. It was different to losing a brother or a father in that I only had hopes and expectations to grieve for, not memories. But this did not lessen the intensity.

We found out that Paul had osteogenesis imperfecta. It was caused by a recessive gene and we had a one in four chance of recurrence in subsequent pregnancies.

We went through the trauma of blaming everyone, we looked back in our family trees for any case where we could find a link such as the early onset of deafness. Both our families denied it was their genes that could have been at fault – it caused much upset. We wanted to find an answer, why did it happen to us? I wasn't coping: the trauma, the severe abnormality and now a recessive gene. People would say to me that 25% is not a very high chance, but 25% is huge.

Prior to getting the results of the genetic testing I blamed the morning sickness medication for Paul's deformities. I had terrible guilt. I had also thought that maybe I had caused his fractures when I had slipped over while skiing at four months pregnant or lying on my stomach in bed – in fact I probably did. He would have been in so much pain.

I did lots of research in an effort to understand what was wrong and why I was not coming right emotionally. You can still toilet, wash dishes and drive a car – all the mechanics of living – but 99% of my brain was focused on thinking about what might have been, just 1% was on the future.

I found that the community seems to give you about six weeks to come right after loss. In the first few days people arrived with heaps of meals and flowers, but it quickly dropped off. The world was moving on and I was not. People stopped talking about it as they didn't want to make me cry. I did lots of research and as a result wrote a booklet, *Grief and the Loss of Your Baby*, in an effort to understand what I was going through emotionally. There was nothing else available.

In retrospect I shouldn't have tried to get pregnant again so quickly, I should have done more grieving first. I was pregnant after four to five months. I tried to just bury the pregnancy, I didn't want to learn to love this child and didn't fantasise about its future. I had lost trust in my body and in nature.

No amount of reassurance would convince me that my child would be 100% perfect and I didn't allow myself to believe that it was going to be fine. I hated being asked about my pregnancy and would constantly respond with *"yes my last baby died, and there's a good chance there is something wrong with this baby"*. It may have been terribly inappropriate, but I didn't care. I worked as a midwife right through until Andrew was born.

People would ask me *"how many children have you had?"* and I'd say four, and they'd ask for their names. Do you lie or tell the truth?

Now, 30 years later, I will always remember; however, with time, the pain lessens.

It has changed my life, it has given me a dimension to my personality that people who have never experienced a close loss don't understand. It has softened me. It has made me realise that we are not immortal and that any one of us can suffer loss at any time. When you are young, you think that nothing is ever going to happen. It reminds you that anyone is at risk. It reminds you of what is important and of the fragility of life.

It has given me a much greater understanding and recognition of other people's loss. I can, and do, talk them through their loss. People seem to appreciate the chance to talk about loss with someone who actually understands.

I often think of how it was 100 years ago when only half of babies survived to age five, and of them only half reached adulthood. There was no support back then but the grief would have been just as great. They must have been very strong women or our expectations must have changed dramatically.

Double grief

Jen Missen

On listening to my daughter's phone call, I was told that our newly born grandson, Jevan, had truncus and would be going to hospital in Auckland. My daughter asked me if I could go with him. She wasn't allowed in the helicopter, as she was on a drip and on a stretcher. There was definitely no room in the helicopter for her bed.

I had mixed emotions. I sure wanted to go with Jevan, but at the same time it was breaking my heart to know there was something wrong with my new grandson.

Even as I write this the tears start pouring down my face. Even though it is seven and a half years ago, the memory is still very vivid and the grief is very, very real. Sometimes I wonder why I am still crying. But as I watch my kids grieve, I realise no one knows how bad it really is to watch your own daughter and son-in-law grieve, and cope with your own grief as well, unless you've been there. I felt like the whole world was closing in around me.

It meant so much to me to have two friends come in and just take over. I remember one friend saying *"as long as I pack you some lippy and some knickers you can get by"*. We had a little giggle. What light relief that was too. I didn't realise it at the time, but that was the last time I had a smile on my face for many, many days. My other friend took care of my other wee granddaughter, while I went with my grandson, daughter, and son-in-law to Auckland.

It meant so much to me that my friends stepped in to help me do something so simple as pack a bag – I just couldn't think clearly and so couldn't have done it myself. My mind was a blur. My friends' help was just what I needed, although I didn't know that at the time. I was completely stunned for those first few hours on comprehending all this, and trying to cope with being there for my kids.

At the end of that day we got the verdict. What we thought would have been put right by an operation was not going to happen. No operation could be of any assistance as Jevan's little heart was far beyond repair. It was certainly a very complicated situation, he had many heart defects.

For me, the reality of the seriousness of the diagnosis was the hardest part of all my grief! I now wanted to burst into tears as noisily as I possibly could. But instead I tried to stay strong for my kids.

I was crying within and without. I can't explain, but I felt like my own heart was going to come out through my chest. I had question after question, but I couldn't even speak them out. The grief was overwhelming.

The doctor asked if we had any questions. *"Yes"* I wanted to say, but I wasn't capable of even speaking at the time. All I could think was that *"I have to take this all in because the parents of our Jevan may not remember all the doctor said"*. He also used some medical jargon which I knew the kids wouldn't understand and would ask about afterwards.

I was trying to scribble down, through my tears, everything that the doctor said. I couldn't see what I was writing. I had to just go by memory of what I'd heard. I couldn't see the lines on my paper due to big teardrops falling. (Later I noticed that I had written over the top of some of my writing because I hadn't seen where I was writing on the paper through my blurry, watery eyes.)

I realised a mother's heart is so big. Often through early childhood years we mums put our own desires, grief, sadness, wants and needs aside for our kids. It came naturally to me as a mum to just want to be there for my kids, their needs were more important than mine. My job now was to be strong for them. This in actual fact kept me going, to a certain degree, as well. But at the same time, I would cry myself to sleep every night, out of their sight.

When I saw our little Jevan lying there, big, bouncy and chubby, looking like nothing was wrong with him, it was so hard to believe he was going to die. When we saw the little wee tiny babies fighting for their lives in the baby intensive care unit, the wee fragile weak tiny things, one could comprehend that they may not make it, but to see our bonny boy, it just looked like there was nothing wrong with him.

After the diagnosis was given, we were told to take him home to die. Our wee Jevan lived for 11 days. We loved and lost.

From a 'mum's point of view' I do want to add this, to grieve for the loss of a child or grandchild is absolutely nothing I can explain. In my life I have seen a lot of deaths. I had my mum and dad die reasonably early in their lives. I've had young friends die. BUT having a child die, it is absolutely nothing like losing my parents or even my friends.

I can't help but say, I found there was no comparison between the death of our parents, and of my friend who died, and someone who is grieving for their grandchild, because you take on a double grief, grieving for your kid's loss as well as your own.

After several years, I was wondering why I still felt so very sad and would cry at the drop of a hat if we talked about Jevan. The grief was still so inconsolable.

One friend with good intentions suggested I see a counsellor. Looking back now, I am so glad I didn't take up the suggestion. I've healed in my own time, but that's not something I need to worry about. It's a journey!

Grief is a journey where we start to make our way through it. And getting through it can take years – believe me.

Unless you've been through this, I wonder if you'll even understand. Although my kids only just now realise the gravity of my grief as well.

It was much later, once I was in the privacy of my own home, that my grief poured out. I had to learn to deal with a double grief of seeing my kids so very sad. It's hard to put it into words, but any mum will know that her heart is for her children, and anything that hurts them hurts us. So I was naturally heartbroken for them, and I found the grief incredibly hard.

I would gauge that I filled a big bucket full of tears. I heard that God holds our tears in a bottle. I imagined He would need a whole room for mine alone with all the bottles I had filled.

I loved to receive things written down, little notes on lovely paper, emails, faxes, cards, as I often looked back on them and still do. Phone calls were precious, but something written is something you have always got. Yes, they'd make me cry. But every time they did, I saw it as a process in the healing.

My daughter and I often checked in with each other saying *"are you having a sad day today or a good day?"* And going by the answer we either backed off or freely talked.

To this day, we have our tears still. We talk about Jevan some days and remain dry-eyed; other days we will fall apart. In writing this, it has brought it up again for me and once again more tears. But I feel it is healthy to cry it out and not to be ashamed even though at times we do try to hide it. I guess that's a natural thing.

Grieving parents/grandparents – you can certainly tell who's been through the loss of a child by what they say. They give great advice, and put no pressure or questions on you but offer wisdom in their counsel.

Now, years later, his birth date and passing date are both very raw. We are very aware of these days. We don't usually plan anything on those days apart from being with family.

Out of my grief has come a deeper love for our beautiful daughter and our son-in-law. I had doubted that a deeper love was even possible, yet it has developed. Out of my grief has come a deeper love for other members of the family, including my granddaughters.

I remember crying with people. They took me out for coffee, they spoilt me, they wrapped me in their love in that special time. That was GREAT!

Waiting to hold you

Elise Atkinson

The feeling of excitement that, after the months of waiting, Frith Elouisa is about to make her appearance. It's one o'clock in the morning and I get out of the car in the hospital car park. My waters break, all over the ground. I am glad it didn't happen in the car! I am surprised they are so dark in colour.

I look out of the upstairs window in the hospital. It is seven o'clock in the morning. All of those cars are taking their passengers to their jobs as if nothing has happened. Don't they know what has happened? Why is the rest of the world carrying on as if nothing has happened! *What are they doing!* Someone needs to tell them. My baby died.

My baby died 12 hours before she was born and I didn't even know. Or *did* I know! Did I have a suspicion that something suddenly wasn't quite 'right'? I thought *"don't think about it and it will all be okay"*. On some deep level, I think I knew.

How am I going to tell Barns, my little boy, who has been so looking forward to Frith coming? He has put all of his old toys into her bedroom. He is at my parents' place. At eight o'clock in the morning I ring my sister and ask her to get him dressed and bring him into the hospital to see his little sister. My parents are concerned and come on the line asking me if I think that is a good idea, and I reassure them, yes, it is a good idea. It is the right way to tell him.

An hour later my sister arrives with my three-year-old son, and leaves us together.

He is excited to be seeing Frith, but I say to him *"hon, I have something sad to tell you"*. He looks at me. He looks at the little bundle I am holding in my arms, and I tell him that our darling Frith has died, and that she can come home to our house for only a few days. He knows what it means to die, but he doesn't know what it *means* to die.

We sit on the bed with Frith, and he wants to see her feet, and her hands. And her legs. And her ears. And touch her and hold her. He tells me she is too cold now so we need to wrap her up again. We talk to her and about her for almost an hour, and I see it begin to dawn on him that she isn't moving or responding. And he finally understands. I can see the sadness in his little face, and in his eyes as he looks at me and sees my own sadness.

When Frith was first born everyone in the room was silent, all of us holding our breath willing this perfect little girl to breathe. That was all she had to do, just take one breath … how hard can that be … just one breath and it will be okay … but she didn't. She didn't. I wanted to breathe air into her and it would be all right.

I remember my dad standing next to me looking at me and tears silently rolling down his face. Holding my hand. I felt so sad that he felt so sad.

When I left the hospital with Frith in my arms, people smiled at me kindly, thinking I am a mother taking her precious bundle home, not knowing she had passed away. *How can they not know!* Of course they *don't* know, so I smiled at them and pretended, yes, I am a mother taking my new baby home. And yes she is my precious bundle.

I didn't have to use the car seat for newborns. I sensed my own mother's need, and so my mother held Frith in her arms until we got to my house.

Frith stayed at my home with us for three days. The first night I put her into the bassinet in her room. But I couldn't sleep. Something wasn't right. Frith was calling to me. At three in the morning I went and brought the bassinet into my room next to my bed, where she should have been. She was silent. Now she slept. She was just a little baby and shouldn't be left in a room by herself at night.

A lot of people came to visit us. I would say to them *"come and see Frith"* and in my mind I was pretending they were coming to see my new baby. It was all okay. But it wasn't. I could sense people looking at me a bit strangely, as if I wasn't thinking straight. They were right. I wasn't. Maybe it hasn't really happened. Maybe it will all be all right if I pretend hard enough.

Everybody thinks I'm okay now. I wonder if they even remember. All these years later. Time heals, don't you know! Everybody told me so. I am all right. But I'm not all right. Frith would have just turned 19. I can laugh at things again. I can enjoy sights and sounds again. I can think of her and smile at times. But still the ache is as sharp and deep as it was when I first knew I had lost my girl. It is the same deep ache. It hasn't mellowed with time. I still cry. I cry a lot and I cry easily. (Is it still called crying when tears roll down your face as you go about your everyday life, but you make no sound?)

I wonder when I hear of some other tragic occurrence, where per- haps several children or older children have been lost. I wonder, how must it be for those parents? Are there 'grades' of aching? Can their pain be greater than mine? How can that be? And yet it *must* be! I cannot imagine it.

Sometimes when I am truly alone I release a deep primal moaning that comes from way down deep inside of me, from the very core of my being. It isn't crying. It is a moaning. It is very loud, it resonates and it builds. And it builds.

Was my dad the only one who knew it still wasn't okay? When we were alone we would sometimes talk about Frith and wonder what she would be doing now. We could laugh at our wondering, but still felt each other's sadness and loss. It concerned my dad that I still had Frith in my bedroom, that I hadn't scattered her ashes. He told me several times that when I felt I was ready and the time was right to do it, he wanted to be there.

Now my dad has gone as well. Last year I scattered Frith's ashes, with his, into the harbour. He was there. I could sense him there, with Frith Elouisa. And it felt fine and right.

I am okay. I'm not okay. But I am as okay as I am ever going to be.

I never held her alive or saw the others

Elizabeth Bozley

A short burial service; a small group of four … me sitting on my shoes in the car, and in the pub later.

That did raise a smile! My stitches would not allow me to sit flat on a chair.

A small white coffin, lots of tears, flowers and a hole in the ground. She was born at 32 weeks and lived for eight hours.

Numb really, a bit like an out-of-body experience.

I had given up my job as Public Health/District Nurse; we had fostered a toddler in the middle of these unhappy years. That was a good focus and probably assisted greatly in maintaining my sanity.

On a 'pick-me-up' holiday a few weeks later, visiting Arrowtown, I recall a strong and overpowering jealousy seeing a pregnant woman in the street. I did not know her, she was a complete stranger. I had to get away, could not look at her, it made my loss feel so so great. I mumbled something and immediately changed direction. I felt stung again.

I began to dread seeing these pregnant women. I think now that that was one of the first of my reactions to the outside world.

I did manage to get my jealousy under control. I rationalised it would affect my friendships. I really needed my friends and many were having babies. So I dealt with it.

I felt so angry at the world, and still numb with *"why me"* creeping in at times, and how was I going to deal with that grief again?

There was a black cloud surrounding me, I could not clear my head. I could not get out from under the cloud for years.

I can still recall that feeling 37 years later.

There was also a feeling that I no longer had control over my body. I had stepped into a space that was foreign and with little understanding or help for what was happening to me. My wish for a live birth was still strong but the process was becoming very scary.

I loved being pregnant: minimal morning sickness, ate like a horse, slept like a log and feathered my nest copiously!

A friend visited me in hospital after my 32-week delivery and she was obviously pregnant but never mentioned it, ever!

That was very hurtful, and I felt my intelligence was being insulted and that I had failed again and was shut out of her happiness. That also inferred I was not emotionally able to recognise it was her baby, not mine!

This was a very low time. I seemed to be isolated again from a relatively close friend who had now shut the door in my face. She wasn't able to or would not, talk about the situation.

I felt no wish for her baby. I realised later that she may not have seen her behaviour as I did! That friendship was never the same again.

She did give me this – *"it takes nine months to produce a baby, and nine months to recover"* … that was a framework to hold onto.

It just took much longer … a lot of my life really; the effects are the lasting damage.

My daughter would have been 37 this year.

In all I had eight miscarriages and one live birth. I had a sense of failure, of loneliness, and lack of reason and understanding of why it happened repeatedly.

Neither my doctor nor my obstetrician could give any apparent medical explanation.

In my last pregnancy (my ninth) I was hospitalised. I had to have a sacralisation, which involves getting the cervix stitched on the uterus to stop contractions. The stitch was then to be released for delivery at 32 weeks.

But … I miscarried in hospital. I was taken to theatre for a D&C (dilatation and curettage) at the same time I was to have the sacralisation done!

That was a bad week.

I recall asking for an appointment for counselling from the obstetrician – *"you don't need that"* said he.

I recall telling him *very* firmly that I would not get out of the bed until I had an appointment card in my hand. I told him that I was not going through all those black endless days again.

Didn't anybody understand?

An appointment card arrived; I attended on my own as it was considered that I did not require this help. Six months of counselling started to clear me.

I think that was the first time I had really assessed what my life had become and realised that I seriously needed that help.

I remember mornings when I didn't know how I would get through the next hour let alone a whole day!

I don't recall being taken to the doctor by family or friends. Maybe I covered it up well? It was in an era when you were just meant to 'get on with it'!

I was recognising that my psychological state was in overload. I had a workaholic husband and by now we had fostered and adopted a 15-month-old girl, and then two years later, a two-week-old girl.

I had breastfed my adopted baby for six months, which was of huge satisfaction. It had been 13 months since my baby died at 32 weeks gestation so my milk came in with a little encouragement. While I was feeding her I got pregnant again and miscarried at 12 weeks.

It was a massive boost to my self-esteem … I felt satisfied and adequate as a mother and much more content and happy with my baby.

Prior to breastfeeding her, it had become really scary. I discovered that I really disliked bottle-feeding her, especially in the middle of the night. It did not feel right! Had we had done the wrong thing?

The La Leche League was wonderful, a sane anchor in my life.

With most of my pregnancies I had always had gallons of milk and no baby to feed.

Sanity at last, this was what it was meant to feel like … success.

I recall a male family friend being very disapproving of me breastfeeding her. His wife was feeding their babies, why was I different? I chose to ignore him and his attitude but never discussed it with anyone!

To my horror I discovered that my baby weaned herself! I felt numb again. I lost that pleasure also. This loss was far greater than miscarriage.

It was a devastating loss of closeness. Breastfeeding was something that was just part of being a mother. Bottles reminded me of hospital neonatal units where I had worked – feeding other people's babies in the middle of the night. Not that I didn't enjoy the neonates, I did but they weren't mine!

The breastfeeding was something I had succeeded at, nurtured and it had worked; I had developed it with friends' help and was in control of that one part of my messy obstetric history.

[96]

There were no physiological reasons found for my multiple spontaneous miscarriages. I have a background as an operating theatre nurse and worked as an anaesthetic nurse. Research says there is a known higher than normal rate of spontaneous miscarriage for anaesthetic nurses, possibly due to the amount of gases around from recovering patients that we stood over in recovery! There was no scavenge system for expired gases, and we also used highly toxic chemicals like formaldehyde and glutaraldehyde, which were used to cold-sterilise equipment.

There are no replicas of us or me! No family likenesses, names, stories and family connections to be built on with family and cousins.

My dreams of having four or five children are in tatters. Isolation. Numbness. Devastation. No counselling available early on.

I recall our minister came to visit me. I yelled at him, where was this God of his? What did he expect, where was his God, why was I getting all this pain and despair land on me again? I recall saying that I knew I had broad shoulders but this was getting a bit extreme! Where was the comfort and support?

He didn't see the need to visit or ring me again!

When lots of friends were having babies, I rationalised the envy and was able to deal with that myself. I still visited them.

I felt left out of life, my husband had a full-time demanding job. Sport was also a big factor in his life and he had the car. I wasn't allowed to make toll calls.

Powerlessness, inadequacy, poor self-esteem, depression, aloneness. I think a lot of these feelings are internalised very deeply.

I still avoid baby programmes as they will affect me. Over the years it has dulled somewhat, but it is just like yesterday if I think about it too much.

Two years ago I was asked to speak at a Sands group by a member. She asked me but then forgot. I was surprised at how hurt I was. Ignored? Not important enough to be contacted? It has taken me two years to make that contact!

I ask myself now why has it taken me two years to do that? Do I still feel inadequate, afraid of my response to meeting with a group of similarly experienced women?

I have not met many women who have had anything like the number of losses that I have had and with no live births.

I feel as if I should have got over this years ago. In lots of ways I have, and progressed and lived a busy and productive life.

I still have a picture in my mind of my baby in an incubator, crying and being whisked past me. I never held her alive, I never saw the others!

Grieving for something I never had

Lynn Froud

Ever since I can remember I have wanted to have children. This is what is supposed to happen. This is how it's meant to be. It's the normal progression of life. Being one of three siblings I thought that would be a nice number to have myself.

I got married at 25 in December 1991 to Harry, who was 13 years older than me. He had a son from a previous marriage.

I wanted to get pregnant straight away, thought I would. I felt ready. I was a good age. We owned our own house, had good steady jobs. Harry told me he was not particularly fussed about having any more children but he knew how much it meant to me. I had made it very clear from the start of our relationship that I wanted to have children.

The long journey begins.

I don't know why but I had a strange feeling something was 'wrong'. I had a fear that pregnancy wasn't going to come easily. It wasn't too bad at first. I mean you have to give these things time. I cannot remember the exact date of events but we made an appointment to see one of the best fertility specialists in the country.

In 1993 we had post-coital tests. We were told when to have sex, then I had to go to the clinic where they could see if the sperm had survived inside or not. Everything checked out all right. I had blood tests and yes, I ovulated. Harry had a sperm test and that was all good.

Next was the laparoscopy in March 1994. That involved a day in the hospital, being put under general anaesthetic and getting my tubes checked for any blockages. In a way I was hoping they would find something wrong so then at least we could try and fix it. But everything was fine. I felt relief but also confusion.

Meanwhile my friends and family were falling pregnant. That was very, very hard to deal with. I just cried all the time. People were afraid and nervous to tell me of yet another pregnancy. I remember not being able to speak to my best friend for about a week after she told me about her pregnancy. I wanted what was happening to me to happen to someone else so that I didn't feel like such a failure. I know that sounds awful, but I felt so different and out of control.

Over the years we tried many different things. I went to a couple of naturopaths who had been recommended to me. I went to a Chinese doctor. She gave me herbs to boil up and drink at night. It tasted so bad that I nearly threw up every time I drank it, but I was prepared to do anything. I would always get my hopes up thinking that this would work for me, that this time it will happen.

This was starting to put a strain on our marriage. I could think of nothing else. I was taking my temperature every morning so that I would know when the best time to have sex would be. We may not have felt like sex but it had to be done. When two people love each other dearly you want to make something from that love. That something being a precious gift, a joy, a miracle, a baby. When you have so much love to give, when it's overflowing, you want to share that love. I couldn't help but want my own baby.

I felt left out, like I didn't fit in. As I watched others having their babies I couldn't share and join in with conversations about childbirth and baby stories. It's only understandable and natural that when a group of females get together they will end up talking about those things. I just couldn't bear it, I couldn't listen. I was so emotional all of the time.

I did start to feel that everyone was getting tired of me being this way. I was getting tired of feeling and being this way. When having my own family is all that I've ever wanted the waiting is hard. My heart was breaking. I wanted to be the one saying I was pregnant.

I was envious of every pregnant woman I saw. I would stare at their stomach imagining what it would feel like to have a baby growing inside me. When I saw and heard babies crying I wanted to be the one they cried for, I wanted to be the one they wanted. I wanted to comfort, to hold, to feed, to love them.

1996 was an eventful year. It was the year I got pregnant, turned 30 and saw my nephew being born.

One evening my brother called. He had exciting news, he was going to become a father. At first I could only feel huge pain. It was always harder the closer the person was to me when they got pregnant. I was distraught, I couldn't even talk. As he was younger than me I was thinking it should be me becoming a mother before him becoming a father. A couple of days later I had replaced sorrow with excitement and joy for them. I was so nervous seeing my sister-in-law pregnant for the first time. I was lucky in the fact that she understood how I felt, and after we sat on the bed together and shed a few tears I felt a lot better.

In July we started AIH (artificial insemination by husband). This was just a matter of tracking my cycle by blood tests and an ovulation kit to see when I was going to ovulate. Then Harry had to deliver a sperm sample to the clinic, where it would be washed and the best sperm picked out. I would then go to the clinic and have the sperm placed back inside me through a catheter.

I went for a blood test two weeks later and trotted off to work knowing I had to ring the clinic in the afternoon for the result. I was on a break when I rang the clinic. Nothing could have prepared me for the voice over the phone to say it was negative. I was obviously heartbroken. Here I was, at work, unable to speak, tears rolling down my cheeks, not knowing what to do with myself. I hadn't told anybody at work what I was going through, so I had to try and get over it and pretend everything was all right. At that stage I was dealing with checking in passengers for flights so I had to smile and look happy. I'm sure that afternoon every second passenger had a baby or a wee child with them, or was pregnant! I never thought for one minute that this treatment wouldn't work.

In August we tried again.

Harry was finding the whole stress and pressure of delivering his specimen a bit too much. He had come home for some privacy and my help, and we had the container all ready and lined up. The moment arrived when Harry had to deposit his specimen in the container and I'll never forget what happened next. He mistakenly had the container upside down and here we were trying to save all that we could! I was sure later on down the track that we would find this part of our story funny and it was. But at the time we certainly weren't laughing. It did not help the already stressful situation. I was so angry. I just couldn't help it. Funnily enough though it was with this AIH that I was told I was pregnant.

We had to have the two-week wait now to see whether or not it had worked. This was the hardest part. Trying not to think about it too much but I found it was ALL I could think about. I was trying to think positively, but not too positively as I had to protect myself if the outcome was negative. So I prepared myself; well, I thought I had prepared myself.

I was having lunch with Mum out on the deck when I made the phone call. Mum had been so thoughtful and kind, and had offered to be with me. I could not believe my ears. Of course by my reaction Mum knew it was good news. I cried with absolute joy. At last my dream had come true. The only dream I have ever had – to have a baby of my own. I rang Harry straight away and he was all choked up as well. I was so excited that we told everybody. The next day I was sent flowers and teddy bears and baby clothes from those who knew how much it meant to us.

It must have been a week later, maybe two, that I had to go back to the clinic for a regular blood test to check that everything was going as it should. I thought nothing much of it. I was all ready for work when I made the call to the nurse and it's a phone call I shall never forget. She was very hesitant like she didn't know how to tell me something. She said she'd get the head nurse to speak with me. At this stage I suspected something odd. I felt panic rush through my body. The next voice told me my levels had dropped and I was going to get a very heavy period in the next few days. In other words, I was going to miscarry. They called this a biochemical pregnancy. I was devastated. I couldn't go to work of course. I didn't understand. It was bad enough to go through what we had but to be told I was going to have a baby and then have it taken away from me like that, it was just damn unfair and cruel.

I was 30 now. Still waiting, still hoping, still believing, still dreaming, still crying.

My sister-in-law had by now invited me to be present at the birth of her baby (my niece or nephew) and to be part of the support team. I was overwhelmed. Of course I wouldn't want to miss an opportunity like that. To share something so special and personal as seeing a baby being born was something to look forward to.

To be there when Sean was born was as close to having my own baby as I could get. It was such an emotional experience and something I will always be grateful for. It was two years later that I saw my niece being born and that was just as memorable.

Christmases were hard to cope with. We wanted to be playing the Santa part on Christmas Eve. I wanted to have my kids there playing with their cousins.

We were lucky in the fact that we had not yet spent a cent on any treatment. It was being funded. Our names had been on a waiting list for IVF (in vitro fertilisation) since about 1994. It was now June 1998. We were entitled to two free IVF cycles. So in August we started, once again something new and nerve-wracking and exciting.

IVF, as most people are aware, is very involved and stressful. It requires daily injections, and blood tests and scans. The woman is basically switching off the normal monthly cycle to have it taken over and controlled by the drugs. Luckily for me, being a diabetic, I had absolutely no concerns about the injections. It just meant I was up to about four injections a day altogether.

Everything was going well. Everything was doing what it was supposed to. The drugs were to stimulate the ovaries to produce more than one egg. Then there were the ultrasounds to measure the follicle growth. I remember looking at the ultrasound screen and seeing these huge grey circles and being told they were my follicles and were looking good. I thought it was quite amazing. The exciting part came when we had to have the trigger injection. That meant the next step was the egg collection. I was given analgesia but could still feel sharp pain when the needle was guided into the follicle. I got very weepy as well but was told that some of the drugs made you feel emotional.

The eggs were being placed into a test tube and I could hear them being counted. I felt great as the number went up. Eleven eggs in total were collected and we thought that was fantastic news. Then came Harry's part. I can only imagine how stressful it must have been for him, the pressure, especially after seeing me and what I had just been through.

We had our IVF cycles without success. At least we knew that my egg and Harry's sperm fertilised. But here we were, not knowing what it was going to take to make it work. We froze the remaining embryos for future use and it was reassuring to know that we still had a chance with them down the track when we were ready to try again.

Over the years we used our embryos but no pregnancy resulted. We even tried adoption but took ourselves off the list after a couple of years. I was still devastated every month when I got my period. I was grieving for something I never had.

Our marriage suffered and, in the end, failed.

I am now 44 and there's not a day goes by that my heart doesn't ache for the child I so want and deserve, but I know it will now never happen.

I will always be grateful for who I am, what I have and most importantly whom I have in my life.

If you have children, don't ever take them for granted, cherish them! There are plenty of people who would give just about ANYTHING to have a baby!

The most amazing minutes of my life

Hollie Ashcroft

In February 2010, my partner Alex and I discovered we were pregnant. We were surprised, scared and excited all at the same time. Telling our families was hard. We got mixed reactions, but right from the start we knew our baby was going to be very spoilt and loved.

On 4 May I had my first midwife visit. Kelly and I clicked right away. My baby was given the due date of 28 October 2010. From very early on I had morning sickness. I was so sick, and had so many days off, that I had no choice but to tell my work when I was only three-months pregnant. My 20-week scan was booked for Tuesday the 15 June. We were so excited. We really wanted to know if the baby was a boy or a girl. My son Brooklyn, who is three years old, had already decided he wanted a sister, so we were really hoping for a girl.

During our scan the lady left the room several times. She wouldn't answer me when I questioned the sex and things seemed very strange. The scan was not clear at all. After scanning for about an hour she told us that we needed to contact my midwife right away. On the way to see Kelly, I was in tears. It was obvious something wasn't right and we had no idea what. Kelly had explained to us that she had already received a call from the lady saying she couldn't find certain things and that a second scan was necessary. However, we couldn't see the specialist until Thursday the 17th. This meant we had a very long two days ahead of us.

Those two days were the hardest of my life. The guessing was heart-breaking. We had no idea what was wrong and all we could do was think the worst. The questions that ran through my mind were never-ending. To make matters worse we weren't even told the sex of the baby. That really upset me.

When Thursday finally arrived we had our second scan. The specialist scanned silently. At the end he gave us a summary of his findings. He explained that our baby had enlarged polycystic kidneys which weren't working, undeveloped lungs, and an occipital encephalocele, which is a small hole in the back of the skull. He then said that we were having a little girl. I was over the moon hearing the word 'girl'. It was like none of the problems mattered to me. But then he carried on and said, *"this means your baby will not survive and will pass away in the womb or at birth"*. My heart just sank.

Our baby was later diagnosed with Meckel-Gruber syndrome, an extremely rare genetic condition. We were offered a termination but we declined. I didn't return to work after receiving our news. I was in total shock and couldn't face being around a lot of people. I felt very isolated and heartbroken. It felt like my 'perfect world' had come crumbling down and there didn't seem to be a way out.

I did a lot of research on this condition and couldn't find many cases, particularly in New Zealand. It almost seemed as though I was the only one that this was happening to. Sitting at home every day and crying was really taking its toll. Some days I really didn't cope at all. I then had to make the decision to enjoy my baby while I still had her. She was still inside me and I still had to care for her.

I had to prepare myself for her passing at any stage. I began making funeral arrangements and it just felt so wrong. No one should have to go through planning their child's funeral or have a death notice written ready to use.

The weeks soon passed by and our baby was more alive than ever. She was so active and showed no signs of giving up any time soon. I wanted to carry her as long as I could and give her every possible chance. I was still being really sick almost every day but it felt so worth it to have the time with our baby. I enjoyed every kick to the rib and every time I looked at the bottom of the toilet bowl to vomit because it meant I still had my baby.

On Monday night, 11 October, I had funny feelings in my tummy. Come the morning, I had realised I was in labour. I was surprisingly excited. I couldn't wait to see my baby. We arrived at the hospital at 10am. During labour I had mixed emotions. I was excited, scared, hurt, upset and hopeful. Even though we were told my baby would never take a first breath I remained very hopeful that there may be a chance I could see her alive.

Mercedes Hollie Ashcroft-Scott was born at 1.22pm on 12 October. She was handed to me right away and she was so beautiful. She was born alive and was gasping, she opened her eyes and moved. Mercedes knew that I had longed to meet her and she gave her mum, dad and nanas enough time to kiss and cuddle her before she peacefully passed away in her dad's arms at 2.18pm.

Those 56 minutes were the most amazing minutes of my life. To see my daughter alive was way more than we had ever expected and she made her dad and me so proud. We were allowed to take her home with us the next morning and that time with her was so precious.

The funeral was held on Friday 15 October. It was the most beautiful funeral. I had had a lot of time to plan it and make it the perfect send-off. The next day after the funeral was the hardest day for me. Actually it was a lot harder than I'd ever expected. Not having her at home with us any more made me feel very empty. I cried a lot. Brooklyn didn't quite understand either. He often asked to go to the cemetery to bring his sister home. Trying to explain the death of a baby to a three-year-old is so hard.

Once Alex had got back to work it seemed as though everyone's lives had returned to normal and I was back in this whirlwind all by myself. I relied on housework to keep me busy, but the pain never went away.

My heart feels so broken and empty. Some days I feel the need to cry and other days I'm angry. It almost feels wrong to smile or be happy. But I know that eventually the hole will start to fill. It helps knowing I will one day be reunited with my baby in heaven. She is happy and safe in God's hands.

Shake my hand, look me in the eye

Bryon Berry

Fortunately the local Sands group was there a little over a year ago when our daughter was stillborn. Initially, I had a numb feeling and was lost as to what to do. I couldn't change anything, nor make anything better for my family or myself. Since that time I have had a chance to reflect and focus on what I could do to make my baby girl Tabitha-Rose's life mean something, to leave a legacy and to help others in a similar situation.

The initial help that was offered to us from friends and family was amazing. My sister turned up with all the thoughtful little things that my mind couldn't think of in its blur of shock. I had made lots of phone calls and as a result had no credit left on my phone. My sister anticipated this, and put money on it. I had a lot of little jobs to organise, and with my mind being in a muddle, she bought me a little notebook with a special pen attached. It was invaluable in keeping me focused.

We had very supportive people who dropped in with ready-made meals and baking to help keep our strength up. Cooking and dishes were the last things we wanted to do.

For the first week flowers and cards arrived constantly which was great, but the quiet lull soon set in when everyone inevitably returned to their routines. It was at this point I felt as though our baby could be forgotten. The few friends who made the effort in this time gave great support and I felt they offered hope for the future.

I found the best things that people did were the small things: shake my hand, look me in the eye, and offer to make a brew or share the chocolate biscuits. I did not open up to all of them or want to discuss everything, but the important thing was that I was given the option. A quick text or email saying they were thinking of me, without expecting a reply, was the least stressful communication.

I decided to do a dedication year for Tabitha-Rose. It gave me time to prepare properly and offer others a chance to contribute in their own way. I initially wanted to rush into something, anything to keep busy and feel like I was doing something worthy. In hindsight, after great advice, I took time to make sure I did things properly.

My two aims were to raise awareness of baby loss and provide the local group with some financial support. The dedication year started with a raffle held to coincide with Baby Loss Awareness Week, which raised $2,000. I had several activities planned including the donation of movie tickets, biscuits for the Sands meetings and the sale of firewood.

For me, this was something hands-on I could do to give back to the group that gave us so much support. For me, as a guy, it was about being in control of something after months of feeling out of control.

Death and loss is part of life and everyone deals with this in their own way and in their own time frame. I found I wanted my baby acknowledged: to have people ask her name. I wanted to do the dad thing and quote her weight, say how cute her nose was and how amazing it was to cut the umbilical cord. By saying nothing it felt like she wasn't important or all the suffering was not justified.

Returning to work was hard; it wasn't just about me coming back to the workplace but also about my workmates having me back. There is no denying it was awkward, what do you say? Do you mention the baby? Will this upset them? In the weeks following my return to work things didn't just drop back to 'normality'. I was distracted easily and found it hard to focus on the task at hand. Others noticed I had a shorter fuse if things weren't going right.

One year on and the loss is still with us every day. In the lead-up to the anniversary my workmates noticed that I was less patient with them and quick to snap.

Given the high risks associated with my type of work, grief and loss are given consideration before tragedy occurs. This helped prepare my workmates to an extent. Some of the fathers I've met at Sands have highlighted to me how lucky I was to have such an understanding workplace. I have been amazed at how this has helped me in making me more emotionally available to help my wife.

Tabitha-Rose was a beautiful girl who taught me so much. She made me appreciate her mother more.

My wife and I have dealt with her loss differently, which has probably caused the most issues between us. I have been more positive in my approach, wanting to remember all the good things, because that's helped me. Neither of us is wrong, we are just doing what we can to deal with the tragedy.

He will never play with him again

Still a Gran'ma of two

It was a Friday afternoon. I had finished work early and was looking forward to my 19-year-old son coming round to my mum's house for tea. He was running late so when the phone rang I wasn't surprised that it was him. But the tone of his voice told me something much bigger was on his mind than being late for dinner. That was when he told me that my daughter's 19-month-old son – my grandson and his nephew – had been run over and an ambulance was in attendance.

My mum and I were out the door in a matter of seconds! My heart was thumping mercilessly as I drove to the accident scene, the house of my grandson's other grandmother.

The accident had attracted all the residents of the cul-de-sac out onto the street like flies on a festering wound. People were everywhere! I parked as close as possible then ran through the crowd. My high-heeled boots were no hindrance. My mum was in hot pursuit.

I scanned the scene. It was overwhelming. To my dismay my family were spread out. I wanted to support all of them at once but I couldn't. My daughter was sitting on the side of the road by the ambulance with tears streaming down her face. Her partner was in the ambulance, as was my grandson – he had been reversed over by a relative's car. My son had been inside the house with my daughter's other son, who was three years old at the time.

I hugged my daughter and had a few brief words with her and then went into the ambulance to ascertain what had happened. The officers didn't expect my grandson to survive as he had blood in his lungs and a massive head injury. But he looked a good colour to me and I just couldn't believe what they said. I raced into the house to hug my son and grandson and talk with them. Back to the ambulance. I prayed incessantly as I stood by the door and watched helplessly as the officers worked on my grandson's little body.

It was devastating to all of us when they declared there was nothing more they could do. All hope that had prevailed was now lost, and the reality of the premature loss of a young life agonisingly gripped us all. The mild clear night was broken by cries of anguish, hurt, pain, anger, disbelief, shock, fear and grief.

How do you explain to a three-year-old that his brother is dead and he will never be able to play with him again on their bikes or hug him or have another bath together or help him eat his food again? And then it dawned on me that all the family had to know.

I took it upon myself to make those phone calls but how do you convey news like this? It's a horrific message to send down the telephone line. What words do you use? My heart was racing a mile a minute. Besides which, every moment I was talking to someone else I was away from my immediate family and I wanted to be with them. I was so torn.

An autopsy had to be done. It was so hard watching the ambulance drive off with our boy's little body inside – I didn't want them to take him, we needed more last cuddles. But they did. It was time to go home. I desperately wanted my children and grandson to come back with me to my mum's place so we could all mourn together, but they chose to stay with my daughter's partner's family.

Shock set in. I couldn't sleep the rest of that night. I just couldn't come to terms with what had happened – I had to keep going over and over it to believe it. And then I started thinking about the 'if onlys': if only this hadn't happened or this decision had been different etc. Of course such thinking is futile. Nobody could turn the clock back in time; nobody could change anything that had happened. We now just had to adjust to the devastating reality.

Saturday progressed too slowly as we awaited the return of my grandson's body. I hated the thought of his tiny body being on a slab and being poked and prodded for evidence of the trauma it had just experienced.

The story was all over the front page of the local newspaper that day so now everybody knew our business and we had no privacy. I was glad of the diversion of hunting out an outfit for my grandson to be buried in – it was a little black trouser and waistcoat suit with a white shirt that I had made for my son when he was three. It had looked stunning on my son when he wore it as a young lad, and I was proud that it was chosen for my grandson to be buried in, even though it would be a bit big for him.

Relief flooded me when my grandson's body was finally returned and we could go and see him at the funeral parlour and hug him again. We could dress him in my son's outfit handmade with love by me many years before, and then his body could be brought back to be with family until the funeral.

I had no idea of the shock we were in for when we saw him. So sad, oh so devastatingly sad. We were warned what to expect but no warning can prepare you enough for such a sad sight. The door was opened into a large barren room. A big hospital-type bed on wheels with sterile white sheets was parked in the middle. In the middle of that bed, my grand-son's tiny little body lay, clad only in a nappy, propped up yet totally life-less.

It took my breath away. I just stood, momentarily motionless. We made our way towards him and I breathed again, relaxing somewhat; he looked so peaceful. We all dressed him together. His brother put his little shoe on his tiny right foot – for the last time ever. It just didn't seem right dressing his stiff, cold, motionless body because normally he would be wriggling around while being dressed, eager to play.

Coming to terms with the fact that my 19-month-old grandson was dead took a long time. You don't expect to bury your children and it doesn't even enter your head that you might have to bury your grandchild. One moment we had a healthy, happy little boy running around playing and laughing, and five minutes later he was dead. It was so hard to comprehend. All hopes and dreams of what his life could be like and things we wanted to do with him were suddenly extinguished leaving a gaping hole. Now, none of them could ever be.

You don't expect to have to watch your children bury their own child or nephew. I ached deep inside as I watched my daughter peering into her baby son's grave after the casket had been lowered in. She was just standing there looking so forlorn and I felt so helpless not being able to do anything to ease her pain.

As a mother, I tried to protect my children as they grew up and tried to help them through painful times but now I felt completely redundant. My son loved his nephews as if they were his own and they loved their uncle. This loss was devastating to him too. It tore me up inside as I watched him, a mere teenager, shovelling dirt into his baby nephew's grave. That's a sight you don't ever want to see as a parent. He didn't shed a tear but he must have been crying bucketloads on the inside.

A young boy's body should be laughing and playing and bouncing on his mother's knee – not buried six feet underground – it just didn't seem right.

My grandson passed on to be with the Lord on 6 March 2009. To this day, the relative who ran him down and who was not charged with any criminal offence after a police investigation, has not apologised to my side of the family for killing my grandson. We have forgiven him because unforgiveness is a self-imposed prison sentence. Nevertheless, hearing a sincere *"sorry"* would be very comforting.

To this day, my other grandson (now five) speaks of his brother every day and thanks our good Lord for looking after him.

Much as we miss him terribly, it is a great relief to know that our little boy is now safe in the arms of our loving God and that one day we will meet him again. His battle in this world is done and he has reaped his eternal reward of heaven.

Why me?

Christine Bannan, co-author of 'Be Fertile with your Infertility, Creative ways to acknowledge the infertility journey using ceremony and ritual'

I must have asked this question a million times. *"What have I done to deserve this? Why me?"*

The pain of there being no answer at times consumed me, to the point of being in a kind of paralysis, mentally and emotionally. I felt I had lost the ability to function in these two areas and went about my daily tasks like a robot, programmed to do but not to think or feel.

I was in a state of deep shock. It felt like I had walked into a brick wall and had no energy to walk round it, or climb over it. Life had stopped.

My husband and I had bought our first home and the future stretched out before us, the hard work of establishing ourselves in our first home completed. We were full of excitement at the prospect of parenthood. I come from a family of five children and Gilbert from a family of three, and we were looking forward to enjoying a family of our own.

Each month when menstruation began we felt a tinge of disappointment, but it passed quickly with the realisation *"well, there is always next month"*.

Then it happened! I was overdue and we felt so excited. Time went by and still my period didn't come and we felt quietly smug in our secret. It was a beautiful feeling.

Then I began to feel pain in my lower left abdomen, growing in intensity over the following 24 hours, and I sensed something was very wrong. After several visits to my doctor over a span of three weeks I was given a letter of referral to Accident and Emergency at our local hospital. Exploratory surgery revealed a ruptured ectopic pregnancy, resulting in the removal of my left Fallopian tube, left ovary and appendix.

On rousing from the anaesthetic I asked for the findings of the surgery performed on me. Hearing *"you were pregnant"*, I went into a state of shock and disbelief. Confusion engulfed me and it was made quite clear to me by the attending surgeon that I was fortunate to be alive. I didn't even know what an ectopic pregnancy was!

Hospital was a strange place to me. I had never been admitted as a patient before and all the rushing and noise in my state of shock was deafening. Physically I felt violated, and spiritually I felt insulted at having been pregnant and now nothing. Only pain. I was very angry.

My anger seemed to isolate me somehow from the activity of the hospital routine. I was too sick to care very much and, at times, in a great deal of pain physically. This pain permeated to every dimension of my being and I couldn't do anything about it. When I tried to fight it and think positively, my energy gave out and I sank back into this previously un-known milieu of sadness, confusion, pain and anger. The nursing staff tried to be kind, but my anger was so intense that their caring was not reaching me. I stayed in my little cocoon and protected myself from any further invasion.

This led to my inability to sense the material world. Although colours were still there, I didn't see them. People came to care for me and touch me, but I couldn't receive from them. Music, poetry or words of love didn't touch that part of my psyche that was deeply wounded. I experienced something like transportation out of my sensing and feeling environment and was unable to absorb anything.

I eventually left hospital determined to put my life back together, and although my family were wonderful it didn't help the terrible loss and emptiness I felt. Why me? What had I done to deserve this?

A week after returning home from hospital, I was readmitted. My recovery was not good and I was diagnosed with a pelvic infection and haematoma and was treated with antibiotics and bed rest. Strangely, I felt safe in hospital. I was a sick girl and knew it and here, if anything went wrong, I understood the very best possible care would be given to me. By now, I was familiar to the nursing staff and, although they were at a loss as to what to say to me, they cared for me and showed it.

The most serious point I reached after returning home from hospital was a deep depression. I didn't want to go on living and the thought of suicide was very real. I believe this was the lowest point I experienced. The sickness of my body, mind, spirit and emotions overwhelmed me at times and I just wanted to be rid of all this hurt. Suicide was clearly an inviting option.

Living in a new subdivision as we were, all my neighbours were of a similar age to us and they were either pregnant or had small children. This made me feel isolated and ugly and desperate to be normal like everyone else. I felt I had let my husband and our families down. I even discussed divorce proceedings, as I wanted my husband to have a good family life. I felt a total failure, and seeing my friends and neighbours with their children only reinforced my feelings.

I eventually returned to work, and four years later I had a second ectopic pregnancy, which left me infertile. We had no children and had lost a future. Over the ensuing years we went through the adoption process and were accepted into the IVF (in vitro fertilisation) programme but eventually decided to withdraw from both of these options. I had spent the previous eight years in and out of hospital and was very tired in every dimension of my being. We were then faced with the question *"where to from here?"*

We have now reached the time in our lives when we would be having grandchildren. The naive questions from other people do not cease.

Infertility is a lifelong dilemma and the wound at the core of me still resurfaces when faced with the shock of new questions and situations. The rock-like feeling in the centre of my body has softened into sediment, which can still irritate.

Over 36 years of marriage we have created a good life for ourselves and have special relationships with many children whom we love and who love us. Good friends and family help the healing.

First a miscarriage then this!

Claire

We decided to start trying to get pregnant last year and were really surprised and happy when it happened after the first attempt. We had been married earlier that year and had just started preparations to move out of our tiny two-bedroom apartment into a new home, one where we hoped to raise a family.

I went to see my doctor and did a pregnancy test. She said the result was faint and it could mean that the foetus was not viable. I couldn't believe how blunt she was, but I didn't care, I was pregnant and we were going to have a baby! It was the most wonderful news and I felt so happy. I raced home to my husband, almost breaking the speed limit, and told him the news. He was ecstatic! Everything was falling into place and life couldn't feel any more perfect.

We went for an early scan at five weeks but they couldn't see much, so we went back at eight weeks and heard the heartbeat. It was amazing, my husband and I felt as if we were on cloud nine.

The next four weeks went by. I had morning sickness initially, but that gradually faded and I started to feel 'normal' again. It was coming up to Christmas and I was 12 weeks. We were so excited we decided to tell all our family and I also told everyone at work.

Looking back I guess I was a bit naive. I knew we hadn't had our 13-week scan yet, but we thought everything was fine. We had heard the heartbeat and I hadn't had any bleeding, which I thought was the only sign that you had miscarried.

We went to our 13-week scan with nervous excitement. As the doctor started the scan he said *"I think you need to be philosophical about this"*. What was he talking about? He then told us that there was no foetal heartbeat and our baby had died. At first I couldn't believe what he'd said, surely it was a mistake. Initially it just felt surreal. I felt sick in my stomach, then I started crying and couldn't stop. My husband was stunned, he didn't know what to do. I felt like my heart had been ripped out and this overwhelming feeling of sadness took over me like an enormous wave.

I went home and lay on the bed and sobbed. I then started to think about all the people I had told about the pregnancy and I felt so stupid. I called my boss at work and explained what had happened and that I would not be in for a while. I felt as though I would never be able to function normally again, let alone return to work and face everyone.

Because the foetus hadn't cleared, the two options presented to me were to have a D&C (dilatation and curettage) or to wait for it to come out naturally. I just wanted the whole thing to be over as soon as possible so chose to have a D&C.

Afterwards we asked for the remains so we could bury them in our garden. I didn't want to think of it being discarded; to me it was still our baby, part of us. I tied a ribbon on the tree we buried it under and thought of our baby's soul being at peace.

Friends and colleagues sent flowers and the house started to look like someone had died, and I guess in a way someone had. I shut myself off from everyone, I couldn't even talk to shopkeepers when I was out or answer the phone. For several weeks I wouldn't listen to music on the radio, it just felt wrong. I had such an overwhelming feeling of sadness like a black cloud hanging over me. I felt empty. It wasn't just our baby that had died, it was our dream for the future. We had begun to make so many plans for our new family and it had all been taken from us.

After two weeks at home I returned to work. That first day was agonisingly hard. I couldn't stop crying but I didn't care. I walked around like a zombie. I work at a hospital and it felt like everywhere I looked there were babies or pregnant women. In some ways it was like a cruel trick being played on me, like being forced to look at something unbearable.

Some colleagues at work would put a gentle hand on my shoulder, others acted uncomfortable not knowing what to say – pretending like nothing had even happened. Not one person actually talked to me about the miscarriage – it was the huge elephant in the room that everyone was trying to ignore.

After several more weeks things felt like they might start to get better, but then I had a call from my obstetrician. She said tests that had come back after the D&C showed that I had had a partial molar pregnancy and I needed to come in and see her to discuss it. I had no idea what it was, so as soon as I hung up the phone I searched for it on the internet. As I started to read a panic set in. I was seeing words such as cancer and chemotherapy. Surely I couldn't be this unlucky, first a miscarriage then this!

Our obstetrician explained that I would need to be monitored by the gynaecological oncologist and have weekly blood tests to check that my HCG (human chorionic gonadotrophin) levels were coming down, as molar pregnancies can be premalignant and persistent molar pregnancies can turn into cancer.

Initially we thought that we might have to wait a few months before trying to conceive again, but the specialist told us not to get pregnant for another eight months. When I heard this I burst into tears, it felt like I was being told that I had miscarried all over again. The specialist continued talking about what we had to do over the next few months, but I wasn't listening, all I could think about was this agonisingly long wait before we could start trying again. I was devastated. I felt like I was on the floor and someone was kicking me again.

Every week I had to have blood tests and each time felt like a new wound was being cut into my heart. Like a constant reminder of what had happened, not letting me get on with my life. Those eight months stretched out ahead of us and felt like years.

I began to feel depressed. I started to lose hope and couldn't find joy in anything I did; I would spontaneously burst into tears for no reason at all. Friends and colleagues still acted as if nothing had happened. When one of them became pregnant she was obviously uncomfortable telling me her news. I tried to act happy for her, but I just felt angry and jealous. I was invited to several friends' baby showers but couldn't bring myself to go, it was still too painful and I started to ask why them and not me? It felt so unfair.

My husband was suffering in his own way. I knew he didn't like to express his emotions but sometimes it came across like he didn't care. One day though he broke down.

He told me he thought he had to act strong for me and that if he got upset it would make me more upset. It felt really good to be able to comfort him for a change, instead of the other way round.

I thought about the miscarriage every single day. There were days I would feel sad, some days angry and other days I just felt nothing. Things got so bad that I eventually decided to go and talk to someone. She talked about how I was grieving for our loss. I hadn't really thought of it like that but she was right, I was grieving for our baby.

Three months ago we got the all-clear from the doctors that we could start trying to conceive. Because we got pregnant so quickly the first time I thought things would be the same again. Everyone tells you to relax, just don't think about it too much, but it's easier said than done when you want something so badly.

I feel like we have so many hurdles in front of us. Some days it feels insurmountable but other days I have hope, and I am so lucky that I have a wonderful husband who has been beside me the whole way. I often think that maybe our baby just wasn't ready to enter this world yet; maybe he or she is just waiting for the right time to come into our lives.

How much more do I put myself through?

Amanda Clunie

My journey with grief started in 2005. I had just given birth to a lovely little girl, our first. She was 25 weeks and 700 grams.

After I had her they took her to the ICU (intensive care unit). I was taken to the ward, where I was placed in a room with three other new mums who had their babies with them. All I could think about was my girl down in ICU fighting for her life. I would wake in the middle of the night to crying babies and just want to be able to hold mine. I would go and visit her at all hours of the night.

I came back one night from there just crying, crying from deep within me. A midwife who was on that night asked me what was wrong. I told her that I wanted to hold my daughter. She went away and brought me back a crying little healthy baby. I walked up and down most of the night holding someone else's little gift of joy and the whole time pretending this was mine. I was grieving for a loss, but my baby was still here alive.

After many months in hospital we went home. Even though I had my tiny girl and wonderful husband I was lonely. No one understood what it was like, living like that with other babies dying around you.

We then, after two years, decided that we would try for another one. We tried for almost three years. Finally I plucked up enough courage to go to the doctor and ask to be referred to someone who could help me. I was told that I had secondary infertility. I was told that I would have to lose weight in order to become pregnant. This went on for another year, losing weight and still nothing.

I remember I used to look at other extra, extra-lovely people and find myself thinking *"well how the hell can they have them and I can't?"* I went back after a year of doing what I was told to do. I was then given clomiphene to start taking on my next cycle. YAY finally, but I was scared. What if the same thing happens again? Can I cope?

We waited and we waited for my next cycle to come. It never did. I found out I was pregnant. Two perfect pink lines. I was so scared. I kept telling myself *"we just have to get to 25 weeks, then it will be okay"*. Just under halfway through I went to the doctor to see if they could stitch my cervix closed to try and see if this would help my pregnancy.

I never took anyone with me, it was just a routine exam. It's funny how sometimes in this world you know something's just not quite right. I felt this the night before. I said to myself *"come on Amanda don't be silly, everything is fine, why would it not be?"* I was taken into a room just off to the side with a midwife and a trainee doctor. He started the scan, and he kept looking and looking. My heart sank, I knew before those words of *"sorry"* left his mouth.

Our baby had died – my baby, my dreams and my hope. I got dressed. He told me that he wanted to see me the next day and wanted to look into maybe doing a D&C (dilatation and curettage). D&C what's that? I remember asking the midwife before I left if there was any information that she could give me, no was the reply.

Tears rolling down my face. I left and sat in the car and cried and cried. *"What do I do now? Where am I going? Can someone please help me?"* My husband was working out of town at this time. I rang him, he was angry. He was angry at the fact he was not here and he could not 'fix it'. I must have driven down the road. I had to stop, I couldn't see the road any more. I pulled over and cried. I had to find someone who understood.

I needed someone. I came home and shut myself inside the house. I rang two close friends and arranged for Mum to collect our daughter. I turned on the computer with tears running down my face and started to look up D&C, support, anything related to this. I had people come round banging on the door. I sat on the floor in the bathroom crying and searching and ignoring them. I couldn't say it. I just wanted my husband, my best friend, he would know what to do surely?

I wanted my baby back after they had taken him away for tests. He would have to go to another town. We went to the funeral home to make arrangements. They were loving, caring and supportive. They took care of most things. I had to find the music and poems. I searched for hours, day and night, to find just the right things.

After five days of our baby being away for the tests, I rang to see when he would be returning due to the upcoming ceremony, which was taking place on the Saturday. The lady on the phone said *"yes it is ready; I will throw it in the bin tonight and send it over"*. I hung up the phone and cried. Is my baby a piece of rubbish?

Next morning I had a call to say our parcel had arrived. I wanted to go by myself. I went to the lab and explained why I was there. I was taken into another room, where I waited. A lady came in holding a brown paper bag. Inside that bag was my baby. I said to her *"if that is what I think it is, you'd better turn around and come back with something more appropriate"*. She left and came back with a box with a little blue butterfly on top. It's funny though, after she handed this box to me she then told me of her two losses. That's what I can't understand sometimes, if you have lost a child or baby, why would you give their baby back in a brown paper bag? How would that have made them feel?

I wanted to sleep with the little casket, just for the night before the ceremony. My husband couldn't understand that. I made the compromise of just beside the bed. We buried our baby the next day.

I then started to have the comments: *"must have been something wrong"*, *"try again"*, *"for the best"*, *"drink laugh forget"*, *"adoption?"*, *"it's only a miscarriage, are you still sad, get over it"*, *"be grateful for the one you have got"*.

It is not like you can just pop off to the local shops and buy a new one, I wanted this one. I wanted my baby.

"Don't think about it and it will happen."

Easy for them to say don't think about it, how can you not?

"You have to take pills on these days, have sex on these days, your world seems to be to make a baby."

Other people that I have started to avoid are those ones that keep asking *"are you pregnant yet?"* It hurts. I don't want to say no, it feels like you are reliving the sadness of not being pregnant every time they ask you, so I have just learnt to avoid them. I have wanted to have a fork or a fire hydrant on hand sometimes.

I had no contact from my midwife after losing our baby. I rang up and had to speak to her relief midwife. Two days later I went in to see if everything was going down inside me. The relief midwife wanted to know why I was there. I felt gutted again that I had to explain the story over again to someone I had already spoken to just two days before. I asked her if there were any support groups within our town or if there was any information she had that she could give me. She dug deep within her bag and pulled out a pamphlet that I am sure came from the 1900s and was of no help whatsoever. It turns out that she knew of this support network here, Sands, but why on earth didn't she tell me? How could you have something like that just slip your mind?

I was asking for help but no one seemed to be listening to me. What would have happened if a mother had turned around and jumped off a bridge due to thinking there was no support?

I knew of people who were pregnant about the time that we lost our baby, but I didn't want to hear how they were doing, it hurt and I didn't care. I didn't care because it felt like some friends and most of the extended family didn't care about our loss. I didn't want other children, little children, around me. It made me think of what could have been. My good close friend understood that and I am grateful to her. I have changed.

My world won't be the same again – I am sad. I have lost many friends and extended family along the way, because they don't understand why I have changed. They have passed comments that I have gone funny. I have tried to talk to them and tell them, but it is almost like they block it out and cannot comprehend such a thing. I don't want their sympathy, I want the acknowledgement that our baby – this baby – was here with us even though it was for a short time. This baby I had dreams and hopes for. I loved this baby.

You don't just have a death date that you remember, you also have a due date. To me these are so important. They make me sad. And someone else remembering makes me smile to think that they care and they remembered too. People don't want to talk about it because it is too sad; I live with the sadness every day.

After four months we went back on the pills AGAIN, and again we waited. Still nothing 11 months later. I had a dye put through my ovaries. I have heard people say that this can sometimes make you pregnant. This was an extremely uncomfortable procedure. Nevertheless you do it, in hope of a baby.

By this stage I am starting to give up on ever having another one. You just go through the process of taking pills, having sex and disappointment, and loss after every month, hoping for two pink lines that never come, and that feeling of being useless and beaten.

For some reason I took a test at midnight one night – two pink lines staring back at me. I went straight to my husband and woke him up. *"What's wrong?"* he asked. *"You have to start building another coffin! I have two pink lines!"* I don't think I can be blamed for my reaction. Others may think that this is an awful response, but I am not mad or crazy. I have just been disappointed so many times and do understand the reality that they don't all make it.

"Okay Amanda", I would say, *"we just have to keep this one alive!"* Two weeks later we lost our baby.

You now have to go through the grief all over again, alone in the sense that you didn't want to tell too many people, just in case. But sometimes this makes it worse. I just wanted to scream out *"I lost my baby"*, but I know most people would run the other way so what's the point? This brings up the other baby you lost, and again that hope is reduced once more. Every time I go and see the doctor I grab a little bit of hope back, but then when they don't follow up or you have to chase them to make the promised appointment you start to feel like no one cares again.

I have three children: one lovely little girl and two shiny angel stars. I do find myself looking at other pregnant people and hating their tummies, and wondering if they are going to be good parents to their children and give them all the love and cuddles they need. Sometimes I have this little voice inside me saying *"don't give up hope"*. I have found myself yelling at this non-existent person *"just f**k off, just go away, what's the point?"* With both miscarriages, when I learnt that we had lost our baby I wanted them OUT! I didn't want to be pregnant when my baby wasn't alive.

My daughter tells me that she sees our baby in heaven, playing in the clouds with our cat Hansel. This is hard sometimes. But I know she wants to talk about 'our baby' too. She loved our baby.

We had our anniversary last month, we lit a candle and we had a little party for our baby. We sang *Happy Birthday* and she got to blow out the candles. This is how we wanted to remember our baby; he is still with us and always will be. My niece and nephew were there as well. They had a very puzzled look on their lovely faces that we were singing this song, to whom? They do go through this too. I have learnt to have patience with this and talk about it, even though it does hurt me. It is okay to talk about death.

My daughter wants to take things to school to share, but she always comes home disappointed that she never seems to get her turn. She does talk about our baby. Other children seem to look at her as if there is something wrong or they just don't understand.

We visit the grave, and she is happy in the fact she wants to make sure all the other babies, and children's things are placed back onto their graves so their mums and dads don't feel sad when they come to visit. I made the choice of not telling her about our last miscarriage. She is very sensitive and I think I don't want her to go through her sadness all over again.

It has been hard. I know that if it hadn't been for my husband, my mum, Monday nights with my friend, close family and Catherine from Sands, I would have not wanted to leave my bed and would have slipped into a really dark place with no light at the end of the tunnel. I have a little hope left, but not much more. I know there are many people who have lost more babies and dreams than me, but I would have to agree that one's grief cannot ever be measured. It is personal to you. Unfortunately it is yours to bear.

I am a very private person, but I am tired of pretending that I am okay and we shouldn't talk about it. I am sad, my arms are empty and life goes on all around me. I don't want a big drama of 'poor Amanda' and the sympathies. I want to be able to talk about our babies, to say their names and to not have that expectation imposed on me that I should have moved on by now. I will live my life and enjoy it, but I will never forget this pain. How much more do I put myself through, my husband and my close family, to be able to fill my empty arms?

I am the face of two miscarriages, secondary infertility and preterm labour.

We were going to play games together

Kathleen Clunie aged 5½

My name is Kathleen and I was going to be a big sister. I was really happy; we were going to watch TV together and play games. But something happened and our baby died.

I felt sad when Mum and Dad told me. I ran downstairs and hid under the table and cried. Mum and Dad were sad too and Mum cried lots.

Mum had to go to the hospital. I missed my Mum.

Mum says our baby will always be with us in our hearts and in the first star that shines at night. But I think I would have liked my brother instead of a star.

Agony at loss of innocent little lives

Anna

In March 2000 I had my first miscarriage. I was alone and only 13. The baby I had been carrying was a result of a drug rape at a party. I was so ashamed of the rape that I didn't tell anyone and consequently no one knew I was pregnant. I was frightened.

Every day I struggled between the reality of the situation and denial. I loved the little life inside me despite how it was conceived. I was at school when I miscarried at ten weeks. I remember I got in trouble for wagging a few classes, before I went to the sick bay with what I said was a sore tummy.

The following days, weeks, months, even years to some extent are a blur. It was a strange feeling somewhere between numbness and agony at the loss of this innocent little life. I tried to create the illusion of carrying on as normal, doing the same everyday activities, but my heart wasn't in it, I was broken and no one could see it.

After a few months one of my schoolteachers could see that I was struggling and took me to see the school counsellor. I went to see that counsellor every week for two years before I could bring myself to voice that I had had a miscarriage. This was the first person I had ever told. The counsellor was amazing. Finally I was not alone with my grief. Together we named my baby Isabella Grace. Finally it felt like it was real, I hadn't made it up, and someone else knew my journey and I had a space where it was safe for me to grieve.

I felt like I needed to say goodbye to my little angel so with the help of my counsellor we had a little ceremony. There was music, we both read something we had written and we released a single pink helium balloon. It was a very special and pivotal point for me. That day I took control of my journey and my grief. The counsellor is no longer my counsellor but a very dear friend of mine.

My partner and I have been together just over two years and have experienced three more miscarriages.

Two we believe to be boys, Jake and Morgan, and a girl we named Sophie. Jake and Morgan's miscarriages happened at home when I was with my partner, which is in stark contrast to my first miscarriage, and that really made a difference. It really helped me to have someone there to hold me during and after. I lost Sophie while I was away from my partner for a week.

I miscarried Jake at six weeks on the 23 June 2009, I decided to try a hot bath to help relieve some of the pain. It wasn't a good idea, as I was sitting in a bath of blood. I remember just sitting there and crying. My partner got in the bath and sat behind me. This was a beautiful moment amongst a horrible experience.

When I miscarried our second son, Morgan, on 5 December 2009 at eight weeks, we went to A&E because I was in so much pain. I was crying and was left sitting in the waiting room. We left after waiting three hours because I couldn't handle being watched by complete strangers in the waiting room while our world was falling apart. The only thing the nurse who assessed me said was *"have you brought enough pads with you"*. My baby had died and was leaving me as we spoke, and this nurse wanted to talk about sanitary pads! We went home and curled up in bed as Morgan left us. There were three of us lying there, and then there were only two.

As I sit here and write this, it is a little over two weeks since I lost Sophie. Sophie lived inside me for seven weeks. She left us on the 27 September 2010. The doctors think I may have lost Sophie due to a urinary tract infection. This is the first time we have been given a possible reason as to why. The doctor also told me that up to two miscarriages can be considered within the normal range. I can tell you that no matter how many babies I lose it never feels any easier.

An important part of my story is that, to date, I have no surviving children. I am weary but hopeful that in the future I will deliver a healthy child. My partner and counsellor both gave me positive experiences when I told them about my miscarriages but some others have not reacted this way. Some people think it not a real loss when it happens so early, some are uncomfortable so they ignore it. Please don't ignore it.

It is just as the Sands motto says, it's 'a little life, not a little loss'. For a long time I tried to deal with the miscarriages on my own but the truth is it was too big and I needed help with it. I have an amazing lady whom I can contact from Sands. She is there for me about anything. From doubts I have about ever having a healthy baby, to days when I feel like a failure as a woman at not having any living children to show for my four pregnancies, to what to do when I have been miscarrying. She is always there for me; I don't know what I would do without her.

To honour my babies I wear a gold heart-shaped locket with babies' footprints on it. I never take it off; it is a symbol that I carry my babies in my heart always. I have received and framed Certificates of Life from Sands for all my babies and these are hanging on the wall of our bedroom, as much as a family portrait would. And I have plaques for all my angels except Sophie, but I am getting one for her.

When we buy a house I will put these in a special place in the garden that will act as their garden; just as if they had lived, they would have a bedroom. After each miscarriage I have bought a teddy for each child so that I could have something tangible of them.

On important dates or whenever I feel like I need to, my partner and I go out to the memorial garden for lost babies at the Palmerston North cemetery. It's nice when there is no grave to still have a special place where we can go and sit with our babies.

I think of my babies every day. I wonder who they would have been, what their likes and dislikes would have been. I take comfort from writing letters to my angel children, contact with Sands, reading and writing poetry about my losses, listening to music that is special to me.

If you are reading this because you have experienced a loss I am so sorry. If you are reading this because you know someone who has lost a baby offer them support, take them meals, send a card saying you are thinking of them. Don't get offended if they distance themselves from you for a while, just hang in there and they will come to you when they can. Allow them the space to do what they need to do. Take care.

Comfort emanated from the light

Jude Bennett

My third pregnancy was completely normal and I was checked regularly by a specialist. Two weeks after the due date, I woke up feeling like something had changed, and I felt quite emotional. I think I knew then.

My husband and I drove to the specialist's surgery. He checked for a heartbeat and his face was quite shocked when he could find nothing. I felt quite numb all the way to the hospital. I was induced to give birth normally. I don't have too much memory of this, except it was dark, and quiet, and the specialist did not attend.

I was not shown the baby's body and didn't really want to look. The cord was too tight around his neck. I was placed in a normal ward where I could hear babies crying and I found this really hard, especially as my milk was coming in.

I remember lying there with tears dripping down my face, thinking I would never manage to sleep. A light started coming through the door. I thought it was coming from a nurse's torch, however it became stronger and stronger, the glow filled the whole room, and a sense of comfort emanated from the light and soothed me. I slept.

The next day I went home. Family and friends had filled the house with flowers and taken away the baby clothes, for which I was grateful. Visitors came and went for two days. One friend, called Linda, cried with me and for some reason that helped me a lot, to feel her empathy.

On the third day, I started to feel very weak and ill, and I had to go to bed. Eventually I told my husband to phone my GP, but he refused to come and see me as he thought I was just being hysterical after the stillbirth. The specialist said the same thing.

I told my husband to call an ambulance as I felt myself sinking through the bed and felt I was going to die. Upon arrival at the hospital I was immediately given a D&C (dilatation and curettage), as part of the afterbirth was still inside, and it was poisoning me.

After going home, I went into a strange mental state of denial, pretending all of this had never happened. I couldn't face seeing the baby at the funeral parlour.

I had a very vivid dream – I was shown three white carnations, the picture was imprinted into my mind.

The next day my daughter, who was seven at the time, picked out three white carnations from all the flowers in the house and placed them in a vase in my bedroom. This to me was a message, and my interpretation was that, even though one child had died, I still had three children.

I then felt strong enough to go and see the body at the undertakers. When I saw my son's name on the door I experienced the first shot of grief. On seeing the perfect little body I completely broke down, wailing and keening. I could feel my solar plexus being massaged by this outpouring of grief. This broke through my strange mental state and I was able to accept what had happened.

I do wish someone had thought to take a photograph of the baby. I also regret not being more aware of the grief my husband would have been experiencing.

Eventually we held a Buddhist ceremony for the family and the ashes were placed in a stream.

I didn't fit in – anywhere

Jenny Douché

After I had my son, Matthew, I had this wonderful new life, I had great 'mother' friends that I met with weekly. I belonged. The Thursday get-together with my antenatal group was the highlight of my week. We were a bunch of mostly 30-something interesting and clever women who were besotted with our new babies. We talked, ate cake and drank coffee, and it was great. We had all had good careers up until then and were happy with our new place in life.

Around October 2007, when Matthew had just turned one, I got pregnant with James. I was excited, but somehow felt it was too soon to celebrate as I'd just had a miscarriage. One other person in our group was also pregnant, and another two got pregnant soon after. It seemed we were in it together. Soon we were all to have two wonderful children.

I had recently sold my publishing business and I was really looking forward to being a busy mum of two. The children would have been about 21 months apart, which I thought was ideal. My brother Peter and I were 18 months apart, and although we fought constantly when we were young, it was a strong relationship – we loved each other.

Peter had died a few months earlier, on Easter Sunday 2007. He was working under his house installing under-floor insulation and was electrocuted. Matthew was six months old. It was absolutely devastating. Peter had been my buddy all my life, I had not known a day without him being alive, now he was gone.

Before Peter died I had always felt that nothing bad would ever happen; there had been lots of close calls, but everything always turned out all right. That all changed after that Easter Sunday. I now felt so vulnerable. The possibility that something could happen to me, my husband, my son or my unborn child was so real. My innocence was extinguished.

In February 2008 we went in for the 12-week scan. Soon after, my midwife phoned to say that our baby had a one in 12 chance of having Down syndrome. His nuchal fold was thick, 3.4mm, it should be less than 2mm. I had a CVS (chorionic villus sampling) procedure followed by a nervous wait for the results.

The following Thursday, while at my beloved antenatal group, I got the news that all was fine. What a huge relief. We could now carry on with a normal pregnancy. The test also confirmed what I already instinctively knew, that our baby was a boy.

I had two months of being blissfully pregnant. The morning sickness had gone and I was growing. I felt the baby move at about 15 weeks. I was happy.

At 20 weeks we had another scan. It showed that his long bones (legs and arms) were on the short side. One of his feet also looked unusual. I was stunned – and in denial.

The next scan was an agonising five weeks away. I analysed the previous scans intensely. I compared all of the baby's measurements with Matthew's scans from the same gestation and researched incessantly on the internet. I became a bit of an expert on bone length ratios and growth rates. I had hope. Perhaps the sonographer had measured the bones from the wrong points, what if we go to another sonographer to do it instead?

The next scan was worse. Both his hands and feet looked funny too. Hope was fading.

During this time I was trying to keep myself busy. I would go to the park with Matthew a lot, but found myself being obsessed with the legs and feet of other children. It would be the first thing that I would check out. I would feel so envious when I saw that they were normal. But then I had to remind myself that I too had a child with normal limbs, not that it helped much. It just seemed so unfair.

Life was going to be tough, but we were going to be okay. I knew that I would have to start preparing myself early for having a disabled child. I wanted to deal with as much of the grief as I could now, so that when he came I would be able to focus on loving him. I met with CCS and with Parent to Parent, a support group of parents of disabled children. It was very difficult, but I was coping the only way I knew how, to extra-prepare – and to cry and cry. I was also deep in grief. I was grieving for the healthy child, one that would run around and play. The future was terrifying, but we, as a family, would be okay – we had no choice.

At the next scan the results were worse again. My baby, James, died about a week later. I gave birth to his lifeless body on 23 May 2008.

Giving birth is hard enough when you are having a live baby, but at least it is a natural pain and you have something amazing to look forward to. Being induced and giving birth to a dead baby is completely different. In the minutes before James was born I absolutely gave up. The contractions were so intense and I was absolutely terrified. My willpower completely vanished and I begged my poor midwife to put an end to it. I just could not go on. For me it was absolutely the worst combination of physical and mental pain imaginable.

The next day I went home. I hid inside for about ten days, too terrified to see anyone. My mother stayed, which helped, and my husband took a week off work. I pretty much stayed in bed, read books on baby loss and cried. All this was affecting my son Matthew terribly. He was grumpy and wouldn't sleep. This made me feel worse; how was I going to cope on my own with a non-sleeping toddler when all I needed was to rest and to withdraw into myself? I knew his behaviour was a direct result of my grief. I had to get my act together and put on a happy face. This seemed nearly impossible – I had lost my brother and then my son, it was so unfair.

What I wasn't ready for was the pain of seeing my 'mother' friends again. I could not bear to be around babies, or any younger siblings – no matter whom they belonged to. In my mind I no longer fitted with them, I was broken.

My antenatal group friends were just so wonderful and patient with me. At my insistence, they continued to send me the emails with details of where each weekly meeting was to be. I imagined what it would be like to be there, and longed for the day when I could return with a new baby.

I vividly remember the joint second birthday party for our antenatal group firstborns. It was held upstairs at a community hall. I arrived late and sat at the bottom of the stairs, crying, too scared to go in. Eventually I did venture up the stairs and then sat in the corner and cried while my lovely friends brought me food and wine, the latter of which I downed rather quickly. They were so kind to me. I had so much guilt, and so much grief. It was harrowing. I remember seeing some of the fathers lovingly hold their new babies, that was just too much. My husband's lap was bare.

I became obsessed with getting pregnant again. I thought about it constantly. However, I was in such a bad state emotionally that I didn't think it could happen. Why would my body let me bring new life to a mind that was so damaged?

Everyone around me seemed to be getting pregnant and I soon realised now that my group of 'safe', non-pregnant friends was diminishing fast. I needed to start seeing some people soon and deal with my issues. Otherwise I was going to sink deeper into the dark hole that was surrounding me on all sides. I made myself visit a baby, but it made things worse.

About six months after losing James I concluded that I was depressed. I had a big black cloud hanging over me. Everyone I met had to know about my losses – which was not always appropriate. I needed help and so I turned to hypnotherapy, with success. The black cloud disappeared inside an hour, replaced with a lovely vision of my brother cradling James in his arms while standing in a tranquil garden.

Soon came the lead-up to the burial of James' ashes, at his one-year anniversary. I decided early on to try and make it a positive and happy day. My husband and I collected about 25 river stones and had them engraved with James' name and birthday. With them came a little card asking people if they could take a stone on their travels and leave it somewhere they think a little boy might like to go one day.

The immortality of the stones meant that James' legacy would surpass all our lives, living longer than any of us.

In the weeks before the burial I was feeling very anxious. On the day of the burial I actually forgot to take the ashes with us; luckily we remembered once we were about 500 metres down the road. I think I was really worried about letting go – for the past year the ashes had been sitting in what would have been James' bedroom, surrounded by toys, cards and other mementoes.

The burial of the ashes turned out to be one of the best days of my life. This was completely unexpected. I realised that it was the ultimate sign of respect to my son – to have him buried like everyone else who has died. His ashes were safe forever and immortalised. He had a grave – he was a real person. But perhaps the biggest thing was that he was now in a public place, a place where anyone could go to pay their respects or to just look and wonder about him. He was no longer just ours; he belonged to everyone and the world.

I started working again soon after James died. It was a hugely satisfying job and I loved it. However, it involved a lot of public speaking and I'd always found this extremely nerve-wracking – my heart used to thump so vigorously that I was sure everyone could see it. However, whenever I had to present post-James I was as calm as ever, it did not faze me at all. It was an unexpected and totally welcome benefit. My only conclusion is that, with the great trauma I had experienced, that my 'fear dial' was turned up so high that nothing as trivial as public speaking even comes close.

It is now nearly three years later and we have 20-month-old Sarah in our lives.

I am a much better person for my losses. I live more in the moment. I am no longer obsessively driven to achieve. I do want to achieve, but only in ways that are truly meaningful. I am very content to be a mum at home and relish time with my family. If we are alive and healthy, then what could possibly be bad?

Insensitivity and clichés

Anonymous

I know that I can cope with the IVF daily injections, scans and all the other invasive treatments but I struggle to cope with the clichés that people shower you with when you miscarry a baby.

We married in 2003. After spending a few years together and travelling, we decided to start trying for a family at the beginning of 2006. We were pleasantly surprised when I became pregnant in the first month of trying. Sadly this ended in a missed miscarriage, where the body keeps the dead foetus. Since that time I have had two more miscarriages, ovarian cancer which resulted in my left ovary being removed, and two complete cycles of assisted IVF (in vitro fertilisation).

After my first miscarriage I became depressed, but I did not recognise the initial signs and continued on with life as normal. I was fine until there was a trigger, then things would start to go downhill very quickly. It wasn't until a couple of years afterwards, when I looked back, that I finally admitted what I had.

After each of the miscarriages, I would slip back down again and would have to try really hard to not fall into the same dark place again. To get through the hardest times I had a dream world where everything was perfect and I would want to go there to live. This would ease the hurt, but reality kept crashing into this world, and I finally had to step out of it and start living in the now.

Over this period of time my two siblings, cousins, workmates and friends had children. This was extremely hard as all I wanted was to experience the excitement of bringing my own child into the world. I was envious. I was in constant fear of questions being asked about us having children and when we would start. They were very difficult questions for me to answer – depending on exactly where I was within the IVF cycle, and whether I had just had a recent miscarriage. It also depended on the mood I was in and how nosey the asking person was. Some people feel entitled to know exactly what you are doing about having a family – even if I have just met them.

Going through IVF is a huge hurdle – mentally, physically and emotionally – and it seemed that the more I focused on becoming pregnant, the harder it became. During the times when I was on the IVF drugs, I found that I would need to pick social occasions carefully – being in a room with pregnant women or new mothers was too much to bear.

We have met many couples who have put themselves through IVF – some with success and some without – especially when we went through the adoption process. At times it was hard to rationalise that these wonderful couples could not have children or adopt when there are so many children in the world who need love. There were times when I couldn't watch the television when they were reporting about the abuse or abandonment of children.

We signed up for adoption. This was a major hurdle that I had to come to terms with, as it was a declaration to ourselves that we may not be able to have a child of our own (and live up to societal expectations). We were in the adoption pool for nearly two years, and in the permanent fostering pool for nine months. During this time we were never called up as prospective parents.

Over the years our friends have been wonderful. They have walked along our journey with us, and celebrated with us in good times and cried with us in the hard times. Some of these wonderful people have gone through miscarriages themselves and/or supported others who have. We find that they are happy to 'just be there' on the bad days, which is such a relief.

It has been a case of educating some people so that they have more of an idea of the emotional process and why it is so hard to be in the same room as another family with a newborn baby. Their knowledge has grown over the years, but the hardest part was being informed of other family members who had become pregnant. Some people have very little understanding of what we have been through, and this is unlikely to change, but I have had to move on.

In 2009, soon after my third miscarriage, I finally took the plunge and went to a local Sands meeting. This, for me, was liberating, to be in a room with people who understood loss and the absolutely terrible things that people say when they think they are being helpful. This has always been a struggle for me – understanding why people open their mouths and pour out these supposed 'words of wisdom' without thinking about what they are really saying.

Unfortunately there are people who don't know what to say or do when a baby has died. They have not been through it themselves and so believe that you should be moving on with life. It just isn't that simple. I have learnt that before you can move on with life, the grief must be dealt with first, otherwise it gets suppressed and will rear up later on in life. We decided to name each of our children, but most people, although aware of this, choose not to refer to them by their names.

I decided to write a poem about my journey with miscarriages and grief, and how other people's opinions impacted on my grief. It was written from the heart and designed to help educate people on what grief is like. I found it healing and although it took me a long time to write, stopping along the way to cry, I felt better after writing it. I also typed up letters – not to send to anyone but as another way of getting my feelings out of my head and onto paper.

I started to stand up to people who made silly clichés, challenging them to think about what they are saying. I am a strong believer that until you have been in a particular situation, there is no way you can know how it actually feels.

The hardest part for me was when I told people that we had signed up for adoption and the usual response would be about wonderful stories of people becoming pregnant as soon as they had adopted. Unfortunately these people don't really like to be reminded that this rarely happens (or asked if they actually know someone who did adopt and then become pregnant), but they still love to tell the same stories over and over again. This can be very frustrating.

With our second round of IVF, I was put onto a cocktail of different drugs. In October we discovered that my fifth embryo transfer had worked. We were very aware of my history and didn't really want to get our hopes up until the 13-week scan. Even after this scan we were still in a state of numbness and not wanting to plan or think ahead in case we jinxed it. It wasn't until the 24-week scan that we relaxed a little, as from now on it was 'viable' – there were instances where doctors had been able to keep babies this old alive! I was able to spend a lot less time worrying about losing our child.

As the date of birth came closer I started to stress about it, and the stories that I had been told at Sands meetings were keeping me awake at night.

After a stop-start labour the decision was made for an emergency Caesarean. I struggled a lot with having a Caesarean – in my perfect world, I wanted the 'ideal birth' where it was natural and with as little intervention as possible. The night that she was born, I experienced my first panic attack (although I didn't know it was one at the time), which probably triggered my depression again.

As we had so many years on our own before our daughter, the adjustment to having a newborn was huge. I was aware of the signs of depression but thought that this was what the first few weeks were like with a newborn. I started to find it harder and harder to cope with everyday things, becoming fearful and feeling out of control. Thank goodness for Plunket, who were amazing and put me on to the right people.

Now, with the right medication and other cognitive behaviour techniques, I feel more stable than I have done for years. I still have good and bad days but overall I am a lot happier than I was, with our beautiful baby and my wonderful husband.

Our road to have a child has been hard. At times, I thought that we would never get there and I wondered what our lives would be like without children. We have met some amazing people along the way who have influenced our lives with support, love, prayers and compassion. We will never forget that we have lost three little babies on this road and their memories are with us forever. I am extremely grateful for the wonderful support from my husband, IVF clinic and nurses, and our support network.

A fork in the road

Jules Chulow

Time is a funny concept. That one second when we could not find our baby daughter's heartbeat seemed to stretch out, kind of like being teleported into another dimension full of emotional pain, disbelief and injustice.

Why would some entity (God, Mother Nature, call it what you will) want to rob some innocent little baby of its chance to enjoy the fruits and wonders of life?

How can death snatch away in an instant something so precious without you even having a chance to defend it? Death is meant to visit old people after a varied life, or people who drive cars too fast and irresponsibly or strap bombs to themselves for some deluded cause, but not to beautiful innocent little babies!

These are some of the burning feelings I felt after we were 'robbed' of Sophia. Adding to my sense of loss and quiet rage was the pain I could see inflicted on the one thing I love most in this world: my wife!

Like most men, I would lay down my life in a heartbeat if anything mortally threatened my wife or my children, but this was an invisible foe I was forced to fight: no warning, no chance to defend, no chance to go down fighting. Instead just a hollow feeling of helplessness, a feeling of being cheated, a feeling of *"who could put my wife through so much pain?"*

If there was a God out there I wanted to kick him in the guts, grab him by the collar and ask him *"what the hell do you think you're doing?"*

Defeat, mixed with anger, slowly distilled with grudging acceptance (what's the alternative?), are all classic stages of grief. I know, as does anyone tumbled into the stillbirth or infant death club.

Slowly, very slowly, some positives emerged from this bitter cup of grief. Like watching the unbelievable strength entwined with tenderness of my wife. Her awesome way of holding our daughter for the hours after her birth added another dimension to my understanding of this complex thing we label *life*!

The beautiful photos and mementoes we have of our daughter (who will NEVER be forgotten) and the fantastic nine months we were privileged to be her parents (some couples sadly never have this experience due to no fault of their own) will remain with us forever.

The way our friends and family honoured both our loss and the short life of our wee angel, whom we were all so looking forward to welcoming into our fold. Friends in need are friends indeed to be sure!

Sophia – one year later – now seems to be a gift that just keeps on giving! She has taught me to appreciate the real things in life, she has made me far more aware of the fragility and priceless gift of life, she has added a much deeper dimension to the strength of my marriage, and she has made me look with wonder at the innocence of childhood. Not bad for a little girl who only spent one day in the big bad world: for me she was an earth-shaker.

We are now pregnant with our second child, a boy, called Flynn. He is a potent symbol of how nature bestows with one hand but takes with another.

With the help of some guiding angels (they are everywhere, the trick is to spot them) we are rebuilding our lives, and taking a huge negative and slowly turning it into positives. This is the very least we can do for our special little girl; she and her wise mother would have it no other way.

I will leave you with this thought: I want people to reflect on the loss of life. I want them to reflect on what it means in terms of the loss of innocence.

Sophia was our fork in the road: one way led to anger, recrimination and impotence, the other to empowerment, gratitude and wonder. The latter is hard to find and take at the beginning of loss, but in the long run pays far more handsome dividends.

Mum is now my foster child

Ruth

Years ago I worked with a young secretary. She had a miscarriage, which was very sad because she had just announced her pregnancy. She had one trouble after another, many tears, and she wasn't the same afterwards. I used to talk to her while we were in the photocopy room. I knew that she needed to talk and that she had been through a terrible ordeal. I decided that if I got pregnant I wouldn't tell anyone until it was obvious.

In April 2006 I was pregnant after a year of marriage. My immediate family and aunts attended my cousin's wedding with me. No one suspected my news, which I was desperately trying to keep secret. After Mum went home I told my husband Richard the news. We went out to Newmarket to mark the occasion. Then it was my 35th birthday.

By God's grace I was at home with Richard when my first miscarriage happened. We were in Auckland and an after hours woman doctor was nearby.

A week later at 4am on Saturday I had bad stomach pain. We went off to the after hours clinic again, and found out that the miscarriage was incomplete and I would need a D&C (dilatation and curettage). I was fortunate to have received treatment from my gynaecologist whom I've known for ten years.

Over time I gradually felt less nauseous and tired, but I was deeply upset. I thought about my loss almost all the time and felt awful. I knew that Mum had had a miscarriage at about my age, and I knew I needed to get pregnant again soon or my chances wouldn't be good.

Four months later I was pregnant. I told Richard straight away. This pregnancy was better physically but I felt under a lot of pressure. I tried to enjoy the pregnancy no matter how long it lasted, but it was an uphill battle.

On Tuesday afternoon I miscarried at work. It was around lunchtime so I went outside and sobbed. It was so sad that it had happened again. I was still suffering the effects of the first miscarriage and my health hadn't been good for months. I saw my doctor and asked lots of questions through the tears, then I went straight to work. I dreaded the moment I had to go home and tell Richard. I felt like a terrible wife. I was worried he would leave me, and I was under no illusions as to how difficult it would be to have a successful pregnancy.

I felt my loss every day and I was very confused about what to do with the next 30 years of my life. I had planned on leaving secretarial work and doing more home-based work. My sister (who lives 100 metres away) and I were going to raise the next generation together.

Shortly after that, Mum told me that my sister Margaret was pregnant again. Mum was very happy and couldn't wait to tell me. I was devastated. When she left I told Richard. I phoned Miscarriage Support, who were excellent, and I cried all night. I felt very protective of Margaret's pregnancy and didn't want to stress her with my miscarriages, which meant I couldn't tell anyone until her baby arrived.

In October we told Richard's parents and his brother about the miscarriages. His parents were very keen on grandchildren and I didn't want to give them false hope. They were very disappointed, and I don't blame them because they would have been very caring, capable and generous grandparents.

In December it was 20 years since my father had died and we had a family get-together by his grave. I wept bitterly. I had lost so much in my life.

In February 2007 Margaret's baby boy was born to happy parents – a brother for their little girl. I was told at 7.30am and I cried all the way to work on the bus. Richard held me and I looked terrible. I cried most of the day at work. No one suspected. Mercifully not many were at work that day.

Margaret wanted me to go to hospital to visit her but I didn't trust myself. I was worried I would cry or try to take one of the babies home.

Visiting Margaret at home was awful. Luckily Richard was with the new baby boy and I was metres away with my little niece. I didn't look at the week-old infant, or touch him. I felt sick and nervous around him.

Soon after, I told Mum about the miscarriages, which was the hardest thing I've ever had to do. I thought telling Robert's parents and brother was dreadful but telling Mum was awful. Mum can't keep secrets so we really had to wait until Margaret's baby was born. If I had told Mum she would have felt desperate; one baby on the way and dealing with my troubles at the same time. I was a wreck the week before I told her and a mess on the day.

Months later, Margaret's baby was dedicated at a church service, with their friends and my family. I was okay until I walked into the church and then I wept. I left the building and walked around the block to release the pain. I didn't miss the service but I felt awkward.

I have had extremely bad menstruation symptoms since I was ten years old: pain everywhere, heavy periods, high temperatures, nausea, eye strain, headaches, weight gain, dizziness, tears, acne, heatstroke, tiredness, over-sensitivity to everything and misery. I couldn't concentrate on lots of different tasks at the same time and was very ineffective. Basic housework was getting done but nothing else and I didn't go to many social events during this time.

I always thought it was to be expected because my mum and grandma had difficulties.

After 20 years of monthly pain I went to my gynaecologist and she suggested tests, which showed nothing. To ease my problems she inserted an IUD (intrauterine device) which releases contraceptive medication.

The IUD worked like a dream and I immediately felt normal for the first time ever. The IUD was removed when I wanted to get pregnant and my health deteriorated straight away. I was hoping for a more gradual decline.

In March 2007 the IUD was inserted again because I was extremely run-down, nauseous and dizzy all the time. I felt ten times better straight away but I knew my dreams of having children were over.

Most people who know about my miscarriages haven't been supportive. They think trying again is a good idea no matter how badly it affects my health or state of mind. They aren't aware of the sacrifices I would have to make or the lack of real scientific data about miscarriage.

At work there was a hurtful conveyor belt of pregnant women. They don't know about my miscarriages because there is never a graceful time to mention it. They know I have nieces and nephews and this helps to fill the divide. Over the years they have accepted my child-free situation without asking about it and the longer I am child-free the more others accept it.

I've had more medical treatment than I've wanted and it can be extremely embarrassing. I'm a conservative person and I don't like blood tests, D&Cs, waiting for results or having my business shared among several medical staff. I was worried people would guess I was pregnant when I wasn't, after leaving an ultrasound clinic.

This year I have been busy with Mum's health. She had an eye operation and has needed several visits to hospital. I go with her just like she did when I was a little girl. She is now my 'foster child', which makes me feel similar to a working mother.

I enjoy going places with Mum because people don't tend to ask if I have children. I enjoy looking after her when she needs it. I phone her regularly and she has filled a void in my life.

Richard and I tend to associate with single people or older couples. I find younger couples with children very difficult and I can't stand parents who aren't careful with their children's safety.

Richard has been very supportive and we are very close. We enjoy reading books, doing house projects and visiting family.

Richard and I experience priceless moments that Margaret will never have, but Margaret has priceless moments that we will never experience.

I want this more than ever

Mike

Babies! Deciding to try for one was a big step. I remember the first time I held a baby, it was sometime in my twenties. I just had no idea.

I was brought up an only child with no other family in New Zealand. My parents were unable to conceive and adopted me. It was after all of their friends had finished having children, and so all of my friends were the youngest in their families. Babies were a mystery.

Still, with all things in life, change comes and with it new ideas. When Trina's brother and wife had a baby I was struck by how the family gathered around the new arrival. And how loved this new person was. I realised that I wanted to be part of this new person's life and, as he grew, I have also grown to know myself and understand that I would like to be a father.

So now we need a beginning and, for us, this beginning is taking longer than we anticipated. It's hard. Each month I hope that next month will be better.

I have a better understanding of what hope is now. Hope doesn't give up. Hope is better shared. And in accepting hope you have to accept that there may be disappointment.

I've taken vitamins, and started wearing boxer shorts and loose trousers. I've given up having a beer. I have a better diet and have learned healthy habits. Sometimes I haven't done these things, and I've learnt not to beat myself up over it. I've learnt big medical words and what they mean when used in long sentences. I've had needles placed in strategic points on my body. I've had to supply 'samples' and to get over embarrassment. And I can say that I have a really good understanding of where each part of this process fits. Above all, I've learnt that I want this more than ever.

At times I reflect on decisions made earlier in life and wonder whether they are to blame. If I drank too much, if nicotine was a contributing factor, whether the Amsterdam stopover was such a good idea, whether accidental injuries to my groin could have been avoided.

When the results of my tests are good, my mood goes up. When they are not so good, my mood goes down. I go over what I have done recently to try to understand where the problem is.

I try not to be angry or frustrated. I want answers …

… and I would love to have a child.

The tree started to die, my heart sunk

Vicky Devine

We planted a tree for you today
To symbolised the one growing in my heart
You were a gift that God planted in my womb
You grew strong and tall, your roots infiltrated my body
Your branches reached up into my heart and mind
My heart and mind were taken over by you from day one
My heart loved you from the moment that I knew I was pregnant
My mind planned and started preparing a place for you in our family
You are part of our life; your future was being planned for

You have a sister and brother on earth and two angels in heaven with you
Your sister knows that you are a part of our family
Your big brother is only one but knows the baby was coming
I know that my angels will be showing you the ropes and looking out for you in heaven
Your big sister misses you and is going to plant flowers under your tree
She told me that she does not want to talk about you because Mummy starts crying
But crying is good I tell her, tears come from the heart and help the healing, and hug her
I talk about you to her when I am in a good space and try not to cry too much
Four weeks earlier your father, big brother and I saw your heart beat on the screen

When we had the ultrasound
You were just a small dot but we loved and will always love you
I had an appointment to choose a midwife, we found a lovely one
I had a specialist appointment to talk about tests to ensure your safe
delivery, as I am an older mum
I told her whatever the outcome of the tests it would not affect my decision
to continue with the pregnancy
A week later things started going wrong, we had another ultrasound
This time only Daddy and I were there with you, your heart had stopped
beating
God had taken your soul back to heaven; blackness and numbness filled
the room
I knew that things were not good but I held on to the hope that we might
get a miracle
But alas not for us this time

I do not know why you were taken away so early, it is not right
It was not a part of my plan but it was God's
Four weeks down the track and the physical body is healed but my heart is
still broken
My heart still cries for you when I am alone
My body feels empty; I used to talk to you when I was going about my
daily routine
Now I talk to you but cannot feel your presence within me
But I know that you are around me
I have two other angels up in heaven with you; I hope you are all being
good
There are also two great granddads, Great Grandma, Great Nana, two
granddads and Nana to look after you and keep you safe, and out of

trouble, and to give you all kisses and hugs and horsey bites ...
I know that I still have work to do down here on earth but I know that
someday we will all be together again
God bless my little angels and keep them safe until we meet again
Love and hugs, Mummy

I wrote this poem to baby Alex four weeks after my miscarriage. In the quiet of the night I had tears streaming down my face, but in the end, it felt good, I had finally gotten all my thoughts and emotions focused. I felt as if I had gotten things in some sense of logical order. I wanted to remember and validate my little forever-baby.

Over the past year I have re-read the poem and each time a little more was able to sink in. Over the summer months one of my biggest fears happened – the tree that we planted started to die, my heart sank again. I bought another tree, it was called *Yesterday, today and tomorrow* and I planted it as a substitute tree. The name ticked all the boxes: *yesterday* I was pregnant, *today* we miscarried, *tomorrow* is another day, you will never be forgotten.

About a month ago the original tree started to show signs of life again, new branches and leaves started growing, we had been given a second chance. If all goes well I will be moving it into a more shaded place for next summer.

Today is the last of the firsts since the miscarriage; I can't believe that a year has gone by. Over the last two days I have been reliving the events and pain of a year ago. This morning my dear husband shocked me by remembering the miscarriage and giving me a hug. If only he were that good at remembering other events! Tonight he read the above poem for the first time, and we talked about things. Tomorrow is a new day and my Forever Devine Baby Alex will be remembered in our hearts.

My pressure cooker of emotions

Sandra Waayer

After a much-wanted baby dies I think the range of emotions that we experience may be recognised as normal; other emotions that we feel can appear alien and often scary to us. It is these emotions that I choose to share with you. The experience and emotions following the death of Kate have changed me into the being that I am today. My decision making, my relationships with others, and my future goals all stem from the new me who came into existence when Kate, our daughter, died on 18 November 2003.

The feeling of not trusting one's emotions has been one of the biggest challenges for me. I find myself making the most outrageous decisions, decisions that I would not normally make. At times I have a desire to run away, to be alone, to seek only fun experiences, to have a day being totally verbally honest with my thoughts to others: to lose all social etiquette. I feel that I have two sides to me now. The side which goes through the motions of daily life; motivated by work, interests, family commitments and the need to complete the tasks before me. The side where others would assume all is well. The side where if they did ask how I was (which they do not), I would answer *"I am fine"*.

The other side of me is full of emotions such as intolerance, sadness, feeling alone, pressured, frustrated, short-fused, angry. Emotions which are often felt but seldom demonstrated to their full potential. This side runs parallel with a possible breakdown of all emotional barriers, which I must say scares the living daylights out of me. This side, I feel, has the ability to take over and consume my whole being should I allow it to rear even the smallest part of its ugly and huge head. I live with a dichotomy: should I show this side all its potential and release its pressure, or keep it under control? I initially laugh at the possibility of freeing myself of any social graces, to renounce all responsibility for my actions, to free myself of the stress, but if we all went about life without a social conscience where would society be? On my happier days, I imagine releasing the pressure and doing all sorts of outrageous things and it makes me laugh.

My world I liken to a pressure cooker. I would love to release its pressure but only if the outcome benefits me, but my fear is that its release will scar too many people in the process. So I keep the lid on.

In my imagination I have released the pressure many times. I have argued, fought and cried whilst role-playing scenario after scenario. What I have noticed is that at the end of the imaginary role-play I do not feel better, I do not feel a sense of calm and freedom of burden. I remain angry, hurt, intolerant and full of dark feelings. The positive outcome of releasing the pressure cooker cannot be guaranteed. So, I do not do it.

Instead, I try to keep away from experiences which may increase the pressure to boiling point. How has this affected me? I know that I do not want and cannot cope with any additional stress or pressure in my life so I do not place myself in these situations or withdraw from them very swiftly.

My previous commitment to developing my career has very much become less of the driver. I want to achieve, but without any enforced employment pressures which I know I do not have the strength to manage or cope with. I commit to situations which I can control. It is not to say that my motivation has lessened, far from it, but I choose what I want to do and can commit my energy and emotions to.

On reflection, my commitment is drawn to situations which make me feel positive, which give something back to those I care about within my work, interests, friends and family.

Conversely, I fear and hide from situations which risk increasing the pressure or releasing the lid off the pressure cooker. I choose to socialise only with people who have a positive energy and who encourage my positive energy. By choice, I am distancing myself from a few friends and family members. I cannot cope with their petty negativity. I notice my emotional distance even if there is not a physical distance. I sometimes feel frozen to speak, to be carefree and to be myself. I say few words, I cannot laugh.

I want to cry out and say how difficult it has been and still is for me. I want to say what little support I receive, but still need. I want family members and friends to remember Kate's anniversary, mention her name. I question whether this is my problem and one which only I can deal with. I question whether I am trying to reflect and offload my emotions onto others. I question how they can help me if I do not tell them of the help I need. I question whether they should just know because they are my friends and family ... I question so many things but have no answers.

I have lost my confidence, my trusting decision-making processes. When situations do not go to plan, I feel an overwhelming sense of responsibility, a sense of incapability, a feeling of *"I just cannot do this"*. I actively go through the situation over and over again to see what I did wrong. I find myself trying to justify myself, to search for what I could do differently, to do better. I feel the same feelings I had when Kate died. I feel guilty about not doing right by her, for not mothering her.

I have so many questions now which I did not ask at the time of her death/birth, but feel I should have. What would she look like, can I hold her, touch her, bathe her? May I have foot and hand prints? I look at her picture and feel that I let her down. I wish I had asked all those questions or have been informed of the parenting I could have done for her.

As I write this, I am aware that time has greatly reduced the raw pain of loss, but my pressure cooker of emotions – sadness, anger, loneliness and frustration – continues. I keep telling myself that time is a healer but I am beginning to acknowledge that it is my loss and yearning to parent Kate which fills the pressure cooker. I seek acupuncture, exercise, DIY home improvements to help release my anger, frustration and pressure, without dealing with the issue itself. I need to deal with this rather than leave the rumbling pressure cooker to its own devices. Has it really taken me seven years to realise this!

Seven years ago during a booked scan I found out Kate had died. I knew something was not right beforehand, but had very little evidence other than a gut feeling. My husband and son were with me when we were told the news, and I heard myself say *"I am not surprised"*. My unsettled gut feeling that something was not right was proved in a split second. We were admitted to hospital the next day to be induced. The lead-up to giving birth was very emotional. I held my bump all night and cried for her. Following her induction I was reluctant to give birth to her. I was scared. I wanted to stay pregnant with her, and was scared not knowing what a dead baby would look like. I did not ask any questions, and I guess this would have been the time to ask. I don't think I asked questions because I was actively in labour and emotionally drained. This was the time that I needed my husband to be my advocate. To know what I needed to ask, to almost be telepathic to my needs. We were very much caught up in the speed of the hospital process, however, now I know that if the mother or child's life is not in jeopardy there really is no need to rush the process. On reflection, we should have given ourselves a day or two to think, ask questions and plan Kate's birth. I wish I could have rehearsed the experience, to make sure the outcome was right for all.

At the time, it was a scary and disempowering position to be placed in. The perceived hospital procedure for women whose babies had died, had a speed of its own. It did not allow time to choose. It was a process of amniocentesis, induction, birth and post-mortem. It was a process that you had to go through and very much wanted to be over.

After Kate was born we came home and I had time to think more clearly, but by the time I realised what I wanted to do for Kate and contacted the ward, Kate's post-mortem had already taken place and she had been sent to be cremated. I was too late.

I needed my husband to be my advocate and support person. He did his best, but I felt alone, alone in a situation that only I could have and experience. I walked my journey and he walked his. But we walked together, albeit on our own separate paths. He grieved in his way, which was so different to mine that initially I did not understand. Listening to others and reading about grief helped me to understand the differences in the way people grieve. It truly helped me to accept our differences.

I feel angry with myself for not making the right decisions for Kate, and resentment towards my husband for not making the decisions that I would have made had I not been physically and emotionally involved in her birth. I feel sad that I did not do the best for Kate. I left hospital with a feeling of emptiness. This feeling has remained. I feel emotionally unsupported and alone in my world.

As a couple we are still walking our separate paths. I know this but I cannot join those paths together. The outcome of this is that we can no longer plan things together because if I cannot feel unison between us, the gap between our pathways widens, and I hate to have to admit to our dividing paths. I often feel sad and lonely in our relationship. My coping mechanism is to not put us in a position where our paths are noticeably divided, to try and accept the outcome of our experience, try not to dwell on it and to appreciate the beauty of what we do have.

After Kate died I experienced some postnatal depression and subsequent panic attacks. I lost my sense of humour for quite a while. I went on to have another daughter, but for a number of years when either of my children became unwell I became very fearful, a level of panic would set in. I was scared I would lose them too, and I just could not cope with that.

Today these feelings are controlled with medication. Today I function well, I am highly motivated and passionate about my family and work, but now choose to take control of my life experiences. I draw away from negative experiences. I do not know whether it is because I do not have the armour or the strength to cope with more loss or bad situations, or because I want to embrace only the positives in life.

I am more than happy to talk about Kate and our loss. I still believe in the beauty of pregnancy, that lots of pregnancies will go positively and that it is a joyous occasion which should be embraced. I would never dream of bursting the bubble of happiness associated with pregnancy and parenthood because of our sad experience.

If reading Kate's life story helps just one person then a positive has come out of a terrible loss, and I will embrace that.

Prayers don't always manifest as expected

Anonymous

Many women want children, but there are varying degrees of this need. For me, having children was something I looked forward to even when I was still a child myself. My major life choices were made to accommodate motherhood, my career, partner and financial goals.

Seven years ago I met the man who would become my lovely husband, and his two gorgeous young daughters. Our fertility challenges began three years later with my husband's vasectomy reversal. At that point I was still very naive and had an unshakeable belief that we would have babies: how could my life be otherwise? Despite that, I remember my anxiety as I saw him post-op; high on painkillers, he was laughing and joking and I was beside myself *"was the operation a success?"* It was, and full of anticipation we started 'trying'.

True to type, I read everything I could about fertility and started charting madly. Sex was timed, but letting my husband know that did not have good results! So instead it was sex every day for month after month – happy husband. It took us ten months to get pregnant after the reversal. Looking back I can see that isn't long, but it felt like an eternity as fear was creeping in. Could I even get pregnant? Little did I know that our problems would be far more complex than that.

When I finally conceived, a huge strain was lifted from our relationship. We had many awful arguments about my approach when I was trying to conceive. He thought I was uptight and controlling and that's why we weren't conceiving. I couldn't understand why he wasn't happy to 'perform' at the right time very month. On the odd occasion we missed the 'right day' I was devastated. With every missed opportunity and with every period, I grieved for the child that could have been. I know now that we were both handling a stressful situation in different ways, though at the time I felt that, because he wasn't seeing it like I did, he didn't care. It took years to truly understand and to find peace with our differences. Now the old cliché is true for us: our struggles have made our relationship a thousand times stronger. It also took years for me to really appreciate and apply the concept of letting go of the process.

I had heard about miscarriage but knew it wouldn't happen to me, so I happily announced my pregnancy straight after my missed period. Two weeks later my smug innocence disappeared forever when spotting started, and so began a six-week nightmare of HCG (human chorionic gonadotrophin) tests and weekly scans. My HCG levels went up and down: hope ebbed and flowed. The first scan showed a heartbeat, the next none, but another egg sac had appeared, looking healthy and promising. The doctors were baffled and could only conclude that I had become pregnant while already pregnant. This was the beginning of my understanding that pregnancy is a complicated game, clouded with uncertainty and often more opinion than fact; that doctors don't always have answers, and that nobody cares more about your case than you do.

I became proactive: researched, pushed, thrust lists of questions at anyone who may have information. By my 12th week the conclusion was a failed pregnancy and I had a D&C (dilatation and curettage). Testing of the 'products' revealed a tri-ploid partial molar pregnancy, a rare condition which can result in cancer. I was speechless! Talk about going from bad to worse.

The hardest news for me was that we would have to wait over six months before trying again. This rocked me: all around me friends were having babies and my yearning to be a mum was so strong. I was in pain all of the time with my need, though I consciously focused on positives and distraction.

One of my worst moments was two years after we had started this journey. Some good friends arrived for the weekend and announced their surprise pregnancy. They were over the moon and I was happy for them, but the pain I felt for my own lack and loss was so devastating it nearly crippled me. I spent the whole weekend barely able to function, but having to, putting on a happy face and talking on and on with them about their pregnancy. I would go into the toilet and crumble, hardly breathing, shocked by their insensitivity and by the intensity of my grief.

Reflecting on moments like these I am grounded by remembering that the reason people don't truly understand is because they haven't experienced this kind of loss themselves, and I am *glad* they haven't. Ongoing loss and infertility is unlike any other grief: there is no point where healing can begin. It is an open wound always vulnerable to more hurt, and the longevity of it exhausts. Infertility is a private pain, still without public acknowledgement.

It only took three months to conceive the second time. We were thrilled, insulated by the feeling that surely our bad luck was over. For a long time I had been aware that my younger sister was ready to start a family, and from my selfish perspective was terrified she would get pregnant while I was still childless. We are a very close family and I couldn't imagine a more painful scenario; I literally used to wake up sweating from nightmares about it. When I called to tell her I had just found out I was pregnant she told me she was too, a week ahead of me. In the circumstances this was exciting, but very soon we both started spotting and the fear kicked in. It is awful to remember my sister saying, and meaning, that if one of us had to lose our baby she prayed it was her. I miscarried at six weeks. Sadly, my losses (three by the time she delivered) cast a shadow on my sister's pregnancy, not only for me, but for her and my parents too.

To my huge surprise I didn't get another period after the miscarriage. Now my stress levels were through the roof, my naive sense of security well and truly gone. I went to the toilet hundreds of times a day, checking for blood. I was in a constant state of fear, which – combined with a full-time, full-on job and first trimester fatigue – left me struggling through each day. The problems started this time with very low HCG levels. I spent a week-end grieving when they went down, then they rose again. A scan showed a viable pregnancy and I was prescribed progesterone supplements. Then followed months of the physical and emotional roller-coaster I had come to know so well. Every bit of strength I had went into keeping this child alive. I took time off work to rest, and struggled immensely with the implications of this. Appointments with my private specialist and alternative therapists cost over $2,000, adding financial stress to the already volatile mix.

Despite my fatigue I strived to eat well for the baby. Every scan and every time I had to ring to get my blood test results caused me so much stress that at times I felt almost physically incapable of picking up the phone or walking into the ultrasound room. To make matters worse my husband didn't understand. The scan results were okay and he couldn't understand why I was so fearful and stressed. I did not have the emotional resources to deal with this. I don't think men can ever understand the way a pregnant woman's energy draws inwards; the way the world shrinks to contain nothing but the life of her child and every cell of her body focuses on fighting for that life. His experience was so different; he couldn't cope with my fear so it made him angry. Knowing that men are different doesn't make it easier for women struggling to be understood at these times.

By 19 weeks the signs were all positive for a healthy pregnancy, but I always knew my baby was not okay. The night before the anatomy scan I cried and cried because I knew that the fantasy was about to be shattered.

That night I lay in bed weeping, then placed my hands on my belly and was overcome by the most beautiful, gentle, healing peace. I knew that my baby was telling me it was okay and after that I slept.

The next day my husband was excited to find out if we were having a boy or a girl, but instead we found a baby weeks too small and with many abnormalities. An amniocentesis confirmed we had a daughter with triploidy, a fatal chromosomal disorder, and induction was advised. We felt strangely lucky that this extreme diagnosis made our decision somewhat easier. This child would not live, so we were letting her go. From this point on my husband was wonderful and we faced the situation as a team.

My daughter's birth, though a stillbirth, was as joyful for us as the birth of a living child. We gazed at this beautiful child that we had created and felt so much love and wonder. There was no grief. The presence I had felt the night before the scan had been constant and real for days before the birth, and as she was born I felt her fill the room. Her body was lifeless but our daughter was very much there, and so beautiful.

The days that followed were also celebratory. We brought her tiny body home and our families gathered. Her nine-year-old sister read her a story as she lay in her little coffin surrounded by flowers from friends and family, who wrapped us in a cocoon of love which buoyed us during those weeks. The hardest moment was when we had to close her coffin to take her to the funeral home. The four of us cried and cried as we placed the lid on her casket. My youngest stepdaughter cried out that she wanted to see her one more time. It was heartbreaking.

The ceremony was filled with love. We spoke and sang and farewelled her and placed flowers on her coffin. Her ashes were returned to us in a teddy bear, which is very special to my youngest stepdaughter. To me, her ashes are not important as I still feel her with me all the time and know she is not gone except in the physical sense.

My sister delivered her little girl three weeks after we buried ours. This was overwhelming and I was blessed by the understanding of my family as I negotiated my way through these feelings. Ultimately, love won out over grief and jealousy and I am fiercely adoring of my little niece.

People are aghast at the loss of a child at 22 weeks, but to me it was no more painful than losing one earlier. The difference with this loss was that it was public and acknowledged and in that way so much easier. This time, my grief was shared and my feelings validated.

After losing our daughter I was more determined than ever to keep trying, despite now knowing that our chances of being affected by triploidy again were very real. We didn't conceive, and some of my bleakest moments were during that year. Although suicide was never a real option for me, I was many times at the point of such despair and hopelessness that I felt I just wanted it all to end, particularly on her due date, on Mother's Day and on the anniversary of her birth and death.

Between those darkest times my natural optimism kept me positive. I don't believe that experiences are random, and through the extremes of my pain I have gained so much that would not have been possible in any other way. My relationship is now rock solid, based on a mutual respect and understanding. My relationship with my youngest stepdaughter, who was especially affected by her little sister's death, has become stronger through our shared grief. In her innocent, open way, she was one of my best support people, always there with a cuddle and the right words.

Through experiencing what was literally my worst nightmare and confronting head-on my darkest fear, that I would never have children, I have gained an appreciation of life. I feel more joy in the beauty of the garden, a sunset, the sweetness of family and friends, treasured moments with my step-daughters. I take nothing for granted and life is so enriched by this.

Most importantly, spirituality has always been central to my life, and central to that is the concept of faith, which is the name we gave our daughter. Through my experiences I have received my greatest gift: to confront faith's opposite – fear, and to maintain my trust in life's goodness even when everything around me says otherwise. Despite everything, I continued to pray for a child and to believe that my prayers would be fulfilled. Again and again I let go of my fear and despair, and re-centred myself in the knowledge that everything was okay.

Prayers don't always manifest in the form you expect. A year after our third loss, we were approached by family friends about adopting the child of their teenage daughter. We are now the proud parents of a beautiful seven-week-old son, and parenthood is a joy beyond imagining. Also, my belly is swollen with a 13-week pregnancy. So far it seems it could be the one that works, but only time will tell.

For now, I count the blessings in each moment, including all of the children and all of the experiences I have been lucky enough to have.

Silent sorrow

Todd and Trudi

My name is Todd and my wife's name is Trudi. We are both 42 years of age. We met ten years ago and have been happily married now for nine years. For eight years we have struggled with unexplained infertility. We were in our early thirties when we first met and so we had already experienced and achieved a lot in life, including in our careers and travel.

Our hearts' desire was to have a family of our own. We have both wanted children for many years, even before we met, and so we wanted to start the process sooner rather than later.

When we first decided to start our family we never ever thought we would be embarking on a huge journey of difficulty with a lot of heartache and let-down. That never entered our minds. Everyone around us – including family, friends and workmates – was having children without any problems.

After two years of trying we fell pregnant naturally in November 2004. That pregnancy was perfect and healthy. At 37 weeks gestation though, with no warning or explanation, our little girl's heart stopped beating. She was stillborn four days later. This was traumatic emotionally, mentally and physically, especially for Trudi as she had spent the past eight and a half months carrying the child we so dearly longed for and had fallen in love with.

The autopsy revealed nothing, other than showing that she was a very healthy baby. There was no known cause for her sudden death. After trying to overcome our huge loss we decided to keep going and try to fulfil our dream of having a family.

We tried four IUIs (intrauterine insemination) with no success. We then undertook IVF (in vitro fertilisation). Four IVF treatments later, still no success. We recently undertook our fifth IVF treatment, in which this time we used donor eggs; these were from a young donor to increase our chances.

After the normal two-week wait for results after the egg transfer, we were overwhelmed with tears of joy to find out we were pregnant after trying for so long. Unfortunately a few weeks later we miscarried. This took us back to when we lost our little girl five years earlier, with so much sadness flooding back in. We sank to an all-time low. It felt like we were sitting in the biggest hole ever and we couldn't climb out.

We have tried acupuncture, naturopaths, homeopathy, Neurolink, chiropractors, lipodal procedure. We have both been thoroughly checked out by specialists many times over and we are both in perfect health to conceive. We do not have bad medical histories. Trudi has had two laparoscopy procedures and everything has checked out fine.

Because we have exhausted every avenue we now feel as if we are in limbo. We are unsure where to go or what to do. Sadly the window is slowly closing on us. It's very sad to think we may end up childless.

We feel very much alone in this situation. People offer support and say that they know what we are going through, but they don't. They don't understand the trauma and heartache we have been through, and are still going through. We don't like how this has changed us personally. We don't like the anger we have from the constant negative results: anger with our loss, anger that this is totally out of our hands, and anger at not being able to do much more about it.

[180]

In life the glass has always been half full for us, but now our ongoing situation has turned that around to half empty.

At present we are in limbo. We are at the same stage we were when we first met – no children. This is a huge emotional rollercoaster, and we still haven't reached our one and only desire and we may never, which is a thought full of sadness. Where to from here and with what result? We are unsure but we will keep pressing forward.

COPING: It is very hard to say what has kept us afloat during this very traumatic and long journey. We know that not many couples would still be together if they were to experience what we have, because of the enormous stress this puts on a relationship. Our love and strength have kept us together. Our will to not give up has been paramount, because giving up would put us in the position of going nowhere, of standing still and achieving nothing. This journey has made us stronger in many different ways. It has broken down some of our real inner drive, but we haven't let it defeat us. We are not only going through unexplained infertility, but we've had a stillborn girl, had a miscarriage, and had many IUIs and IVFs followed by negative pregnancy results. It is a lot to cope with all in one cup.

Many tears have been shed; it's helped as you can't hold all these emotions in forever, they need to be acknowledged. We do have moments when all is good, then certain moments can trigger dark days where a sweeping wave of emotions flood in. Those dark days are the hardest and we need to draw on all our reserves to get through them.

OUTLETS: We have purposely pursued a variety of hobbies and interests to give us an outlet, rather than having this consume us. I've kept active to burn energy and to make me feel better within myself. I've done mountain biking, gym and tramping to relieve stress. Trudi gets a lot of peace and calmness from gardening.

These interests take our minds off our situation for a short time, which helps. We found that doing things together such as watching movies, travel, brewing coffee, listening to music and just treating each other are also great distractions.

Good communication is vital to survival. Some days when I'm feeling down I won't share my thoughts with Trudi, and vice versa, but we both know that when the time is right we will open up to one another – putting all the cards on the table. This gives us an understanding of how this is affecting us both in different ways. We can then lean on one another and offer support.

Our faith in God has kept us solid and carried us through. It gives us strength and comfort knowing that God has things in hand even when they seem out of control. It helps to be able to pray to him through the Holy Spirit. Only God knows what the future holds and his plan, way and timing are perfect even if we can't see it: Philippians 4:13, Romans 8:28

OTHERS: We do know that family and friends do really care and only wish to find the solution to fix this for us. They love us and hate seeing our hurt. They try their best to offer support, which they do with great love, but it is hard sometimes to find comfort in it, as they don't really know what it's like to go through this. You would have to go through this yourself to have a complete grasp of how it feels. We just think that our experience and perspective on the whole journey are totally different from the experience and perspective of those who haven't been through it, and this leads to misunderstandings as to how to deal with it. Shall we say something? Shall we say nothing? All we can say is the best way to deal with this is to communicate.

A lot of people, I think, feel that we have moved on as it has been six years since we lost our little girl. They don't actually realise that we have this huge mountain of unexplained infertility to deal with as well, which has been constantly in our face for so long.

Trudi and I love to speak about our little girl openly, as we draw comfort from doing so. It seems sometimes that to our family and friends, it is a closed subject. Maybe they are worried that they will upset us if they mention her. We get so much joy when she is mentioned, as this tells us she is never forgotten.

COMMENTS: Many people think they are saying the right thing – but they aren't. Maybe they think their comments may help us or maybe they just aren't thinking before speaking – *"at least you know you can get pregnant"*, *"you'll get there one day"*, *"think of how much money you'll save"*, *"we understand exactly what you are going through as it took us six months of trying"*, *"when are you going to have more children, time is ticking"*, *"do you think you guys will try again?"*, *"at least you have the freedom to do anything at any time because you don't have children"*, *"oh they (children) are such a strain"*. There will always be comments that are just not right. You have to be prepared as they can be upsetting.

IN CLOSING: We haven't left any stone unturned in our quest to have children. Our journey has been really drawn-out to the point of total exhaustion, with so much emotional stress and sadness. Infertility is something we didn't choose and didn't think about when we first decided to start a family. It has come into our life and, as much as we don't like it, we have to live with it. Giving up isn't an option. Coming to terms with infertility is very tough as it is always lurking in the background. As every month passes by without the happy result we desire, it just confirms our predicament.

We don't know what the future holds, but all we can do as a couple is continue to love and support one another and draw the strength needed to survive the anguish this situation brings. We look at what we have with each other and draw appreciation from that, rather than looking at not being able to have a family as the end of all things. We will continue to press on towards our goal, not knowing what tomorrow will bring but living in the hope of one day receiving the gift we so desire.

Sadly life goes on and time ticks by and some things in this life just go unexplained. It does seem very unfair, but trying to grasp hold of something you have no control over and make sense of it is an endless road which never gives you the answers.

We have been dealt this hand in life and it may seem like a bad one but we will continue to hold the hope that one day soon our joy may be full.

The longing was ever-present

Mary Clark

We were young and had only been married for a few months. Although I never imagined that infertility would be an issue for me, I thought that maybe we should start trying for a baby sooner rather than later. My older sister had taken three years to become pregnant with my nephew, and I had shared her heartache at having to wait so long to conceive. I had also shared her joy when my nephew was born.

We were lucky – after just two months I was pregnant and struggling to cope with morning sickness, which finally, and to my great relief, left halfway through the pregnancy. Ben arrived ten days early after a quick labour. He was not the easiest baby; he seemed happiest when he had our full attention, and saw little need to sleep. It took the best part of a year for us to get some order in our lives and accept that our child was not like other babies. At that stage we had no idea that our difficult little bundle of joy would be diagnosed at age six with Asperger's syndrome, as well as being intellectually gifted. No wonder he found being a baby difficult and probably a bit boring!

Despite finding parenting a challenge, we decided to give it another go. Perhaps a brother or sister for Ben would be good for him and us. Once again I conceived quickly, and in just one month I was pregnant with Lily. While I was pregnant with her, I completed my training to become a midwife. Lily was born at home just before Christmas. She was a dream baby – unlike her brother – she was happy and content to feed, sleep and smile. My husband Arthur commented that he now understood why people choose to have lots of children if they were all like this!

I returned to work part-time at the delivery suite when Lily was nine months old. Despite juggling two small children and work, life was pretty good. Ben started preschool and we also had a nanny to help. When Lily was a little over two we decided to have one more child and once more I was pregnant within a month or two. I was, as usual, feeling pretty sick but I continued to work part-time at the delivery suite.

It was during a well-earned holiday sailing in the islands of Tonga, miles from civilisation, that I began to have some odd pains. But they seemed to settle down with some rest. On the day after our return home, and after a late shift at the hospital, I knew something was very wrong. I felt very sick and was in pain. Arthur rang our friend Erica, a GP, and when she examined me she couldn't hear our baby's heartbeat. At 13 weeks we should have been able to hear the baby, and although I had no bleeding, just the pain, Erica urgently sent us to see an obstetrician. He scanned me, to find that our baby was not in my uterus but in the Fallopian tube. I was rushed to theatre. I told the anaesthetist (a friend from the hospital) not to wake me up if I was to lose my baby. He did wake me up.

Our perfect little baby looked like a little wax model. We could see he was a boy, and we named him Leo. I took him home in a little jar of liquid, and we buried him in a quiet corner of our garden. I almost felt ashamed of wanting to mark my son's loss when everyone else was so happy that I was alive. If we had not returned from Tonga on that day my Fallopian tube would have ruptured, and I would have bled to death a long way from help. But I did not feel lucky.

I returned to work and helped other women to birth babies, all the while feeling empty and sad. Weeks passed and I was feeling no better. I decided to talk to a counsellor, who was helpful – she explained to me that other people would struggle to understand my sadness, as miscarriage is such an intangible thing for people other than the mother. She said that, in her experience, after a husband dies a widow is often asked at around six weeks when she is going to sell the house and move on. So, if that happens after a long marriage, it was likely that I would not be given much time to grieve for the loss of a baby who was not even real to others. I would be expected to be getting back to my old self pretty much right away. This realisation made a difference for me. I stopped expecting others to understand my loss, and I allowed myself to be sad whilst at the same time hoping to be pregnant again soon.

Within six months I was pregnant with our second son. Other than morning sickness, which was debilitating for the entire pregnancy, all was well, and Darcy was born at home after a 40-minute labour. He was a beautiful baby full of smiles, but he was slow to gain weight and seemed somehow fragile.

I found it hard to describe the intensity of my feelings for this baby. I worried that other people would notice that he had captured my heart so completely there seemed little room for anything else. My world felt complete and full, yet I could not shake a feeling of foreboding and feared that something would happen to Darcy. Arthur felt sure our family was complete, and somewhat reluctantly I agreed to him having a vasectomy but not before he agreed to bank sperm. The nagging doubt that something would go wrong would not go away.

On a cold winter night in June I was alone in the house, the three children sleeping. Darcy was now a busy eight-month-old. Arthur was out at a movie. It was nearing 10pm, and as I was making a cup of tea I heard Darcy cry and then settle back to sleep. I thought to myself that I would check him on the way to bed in a few minutes. As I approached his room and walked in I knew he was not there, his little body was still and the blanket was over his head. I pulled it back and I knew he was dead. I made no attempt to resuscitate him; I just knew he was not coming back to us.

My world felt as though it had ended and, as if in slow motion, I rang my mum and dad, our GP friend Erica, my friend Lynette, and my friend and midwife Anna. I was numb, chaos began to swirl around me. Police officers arrived and were talking to me. Arthur arrived home.

Nothing made sense, I only wanted to be with my baby. An ache had developed in my chest that was to become a constant part of my being for a long time. Nobody could tell us why our sweet smiley son had died. Later, the autopsy found he did not suffocate, he simply stopped breathing; he was one of the 200 or so babies who died of cot death that year.

My life had changed forever. I felt as though I was sleepwalking and not really living, but I somehow cared for Lily and Ben. We moved house, for a new start.

My life was now divided into before Darcy's death and after. After was a world where all the light and warmth seemed to have gone. Other women who had lost babies and children materialised as if by magic and told me their stories. I took comfort in the knowledge they had all found a way back to being happy, they all seemed so normal and I hoped one day I would be too.

We set about trying to get pregnant again via artificial insemination. We were not lucky, and so we decided to try for a reversal of Arthur's vasectomy. I did become pregnant and miscarried at ten weeks; and then again a year later, this time I miscarried at six weeks. I tried so hard to be content with our two great children, both now approaching the end of primary school, but the longing for another baby was an ever-present force. We contemplated adoption or more fertility treatment, but by this stage I had had surgery for a twisted ovary so now had a tube on one side and an ovary on the other. The odds of conceiving were not good.

In the end I decided to try to live with, and accept, the fact that we would not have another child. Over time I learned to live with the pain of Darcy's death. I learned a lot about grief, like the way the strangest little thing can take you back and the tears will return, even when you least expect it. The years passed and I decided to return to university and study psychology. I felt that I had accepted, and truly believed, that we wouldn't have any more children.

At the age of 43, and in the last year of my undergraduate degree, I thought I was either going into menopause or just maybe I was pregnant. Much to our delight it was the latter. I didn't really believe our baby was here to stay. I had a scan with a feeling of dread: it must be in my tube or not have a heartbeat. It was wonderful and strange to see a perfect little baby on the screen in the right place with a beating heart. We broke the news. Lily at 15 was delighted at the thought of a baby; Ben was also very happy, but at 18 said he didn't want to think about how it got to be there!

Our beautiful baby girl Annabella arrived nine months later at home after a two-hour labour and on Arthur's birthday, a true miracle. I had turned 44 the month before.

Now, five years later, I look at her sweet face every day and still cannot believe she is truly ours. Darcy would have been 16 this year, and sometimes I can still cry as if he had died yesterday but I also love my life. I am grateful that Darcy's short life was with us, and that he knew only love in his life. We treasure his memory.

It made me feel like just a number

CMK

I miscarried twins on the 10 November 2010. They would have been my fourth and fifth babies, but it does not make a difference. I'm hurting so much. I have found the whole experience extremely horrific and honestly cannot believe how badly things were handled.

I went to my midwife on 9 November telling her that I was bleeding. She said that as I had no pain I wasn't to worry. Over the next two days the bleeding increased. I started passing large clots of blood and needed to go to the hospital, so I rang my husband, who works nights, to take me.

My husband dropped me off at the hospital and I walked into the emergency department with a towel between my legs. I was dripping blood everywhere and the receptionist asked me *"are you all right?"*

I was taken into a cubicle, then was questioned as to whether I had ever been sexually or physically abused by my husband. I understand that there is a policy, but at the time I was in no mood for such things. Then I had two male doctors wanting to look up my 'parts' and that is when my baby came out. I was 16 weeks pregnant. The doctor said *"yes you have lost your baby, do you want to look at it?"* His bedside manner was appalling!

I was handed my tiny baby in a towel and a lovely nurse sat with me. She was like an angel because at that time I was broken-hearted. I continued to bleed and pass clots so they decided to send me for a scan. That is when baby two was discovered. I had no idea that I was having twins. It was the most heartbreaking experience of my life.

I was taken to theatre for a D&C (dilatation and curettage) as I was bleeding so heavily. I asked for my babies to be returned to me. The next day I went home, but was told that as I was in my second trimester the babies would be sent to a lab for an autopsy and that I would get them back in a week.

I had family members tell me I should get 'fixed' or make my husband have a vasectomy. I had friends say *"well at least you will lose weight"* and *"at least you won't have five kids to run around after"* and *"at least you lost them before you had them"*.

People either say the wrong thing or don't speak at all. My brother hasn't come to see me. He told my mother he doesn't know what to say to me.

Then, to add insult to injury, my husband didn't get paid for the week he had off work. The reason given was miscarriage is not a death so you can't take bereavement leave, you have to take sick leave – and he had no sick leave left. Never mind that he had to look after a wife who had just miscarried twins, plus a three-year-old, a two-year-old and a one-year-old!

The week passed and I rang the lab. They said that the babies were not back, but I would get what was left of them when they were ready. This was a kick in the guts for me and my husband, as we were desperately waiting for our babies to be returned home. Comments like that were just so painful.

When the hospital lab rang to say our babies were ready we picked them up in a brown-paper-bag-covered container – seeing them treated like that just ripped my heart out again.

My husband and I bought a beautiful box for our two little angels and together we sealed our babies (in a box set in concrete). We said our good-byes. It was so hard, yet so healing, to have our babies home with us.

On 28 November I turned 35. The next day my midwife rang to find out why I hadn't been to visit her. I told her that I had miscarried and she said that she didn't know as the hospital didn't give any notes to her. It made me feel like just a number. There was no *"sorry for your loss"*, no nothing.

Later my midwife rang back and said she hadn't checked her email, and then said *"oh you lost two boys, no reason why, just one of those things, if you ever need a midwife you have my number …"*

I'm a broken-hearted mummy who feels like she doesn't matter, and what's left of my baby boys is sitting in a beautiful box in my room until we decide what to do with them …

Miscarriage, it sucks!

POF – practising our faith

Nicole Evans

"Well, to use your own words, it looks like your ovaries have 'quit'."
These were the words of the endocrinologist I'd been referred to. I had missed two periods while on the pill, and my GP (after ruling out pregnancy) had explained that for some reason my ovaries weren't working properly. She had been fairly sure there'd be some way of fixing it, but now my worst fear had come true. The endocrinologist had delivered the devastating blow: I was infertile. I was told I had fluctuating ovarian function, a precursor to premature ovarian failure (POF).

I was in shock. So was my husband, who held my hand through the entire appointment. I was only 30 years old. This couldn't be happening. My mother went through menopause in her fifties. There must be some mistake. However, a second opinion only confirmed the first and we now had to deal with this life-changing diagnosis.

I read a lot and did my best to grasp all the implications, but I was overwhelmed. How could I be (presumably) fertile and on the pill one day, and menopausal and being offered HRT (hormone replacement therapy) the next? It made no sense. All of a sudden I didn't know who I was any more. I felt I had aged 20 years in that one appointment.

My personal identity as a wife and future mother no longer applied and I spiralled into despair. I wondered if my husband would want me anymore, and it took me a long time (and lots of people telling me) to realise he didn't marry my ovaries or my baby-making potential. He married me.

When I finally understood that, it just blew me away. My own expectations of myself were far different from his.

My husband went to all my early appointments and has been my rock through this whole experience. He's always had a very strong faith that God is looking after him and is with him every day. He showed his true colours right after the initial diagnosis: rather than focusing on the family we now may never have, he thought of the spare time and money we'd have and took me in his arms and said *"well, we can go on that big overseas trip now, can't we?!"* He made me smile in the middle of my shock, fear and grief. He still does that to this day and I'm depending on him to continue doing that always.

My own faith journey has been somewhat rockier. I railed against a God who could let this happen to me. I demanded to know what I'd ever done to deserve this fate. From the depths of my soul I wanted to know *"why me?"* My husband was confident there'd be a reason and, although I couldn't accept it at the time, I have since realised he was right.

The NZ Early Menopause Support Group has been my lifeline. I've made friends with some amazing women, many of whom are dealing with much harder issues than my own, and I no longer ask *"why me?"* I have my answer. I have a new and strong passion to make a difference in the lives of women living with early menopause. Taking over the running of this support group has filled my life with satisfaction and meaning, and fulfils more than a small part of my motherly desire to nurture.

God has been with me through this whole experience, and He has stepped in on many occasions when I've reached the end of my ability to cope either with my own issues or with the demands of the support group. These occasions are usually very raw and intimate and not particularly pretty, but moments like these have opened my heart to the exquisite beauty of His love for me. I'm learning to lean on Him.

POF has also taught me a lot about how resilient the human soul is, how it can rebound from almost anything.

Around the time of my diagnosis my husband and I used to do a lot of driving to visit his parents who live a couple of hours away from us, and it was on those drives, where we had no distractions, that the matters of the heart bubbled to the surface demanding our attention. I shed many tears and gave in to the ugly self-pitying side of myself I usually prefer to keep hidden. But those 'discussions' were very therapeutic and helped me to process the vast range of emotions I was experiencing: my anger at the situation; my grief for what could never be; my fear of what the future held. The biggest hurdle for me was grieving the loss of our future biological children. I felt my body had let me down big time, and the irony of how careful I'd been for so long to prevent pregnancy did not escape me.

Getting these negative emotions out of my system allowed me to make room for some positive ones and, with time (the great healer), I was slowly able to start looking at the options in front of us rather than the obstacles. My soul was reshaping itself to fit the new situation.

Eventually I found enough acceptance to consider donor egg IVF (in vitro fertilisation), but this process was so much harder than I could ever have imagined. The fertility specialists didn't treat me like the special case I felt I was. Where was the compassion? They didn't have a guaranteed solution to my problem, the statistics they threw around were misleading at best, and worst of all they had no clue as to why it wasn't working. These were the things I'd expected them to excel at and I wasn't prepared for all this extra uncertainty when I was already standing on shaky ground. On top of that, every day we were reminded of what we didn't have.

Everywhere we looked were pregnant tummies and babies and pregnancy announcements. It coloured our entire world.

We did two donor egg cycles over two years with two dear friends. Sadly, we didn't end up with the child we so desperately wanted.

With each setback it got harder and harder to pick myself up off the floor. Yes, this was the only way to achieve our dream, but the fear of failure was crippling. After the first cycle I even found I was subconsciously suppressing my desire for a baby because it was so hard to face the possibility of failure again.

Our lives were basically on hold, in limbo. Our dreams were in other people's hands. Our financial and career decisions had to be made with IVF in mind. We had to fit into our donors' schedules, meet all the clinic's criteria, jump through all the right hoops. It was soul-destroying stuff.

But somehow we're here on the other side of IVF, still together, still smiling, souls intact.

I didn't consciously realise when I was 'finished' with IVF. I was telling my husband about a friend's visit with her six-month-old baby boy. These visits are usually good for about five minutes and then I tend to go downhill inside. Then when they leave I'm usually left with that familiar hollow, childless ache.

As I got to the part about them leaving, I mentioned that I hadn't had that feeling this time. I was in the middle of writing it off to being simply one of my 'good days' when he stopped me mid-sentence. He got me to repeat myself, and as I did I actually heard what I'd said. It really surprised me to realise that I'd subconsciously closed the IVF door and I was okay with it. And I feel the best I've felt in a long time.

Our focus is now on what we have rather than what we don't have. Our private parts are private again. We are free to dream again. It is liberating to have found a sort of peace with our situation, although I'm sure the loss will always be felt.

I was dreading 'giving up' IVF and the failure and disappointment I thought I'd feel, but again my soul has surprised me at just how tough it is.

As a newly married couple, we desired a family. When we were told how difficult this might be, we grieved.

We tried IVF and failed and grieved.

Then tried and failed and grieved again. And now it's over.

My resilient soul has been through it all and, although it's a different shape now to how it started out, somehow it's still holding me together. I thank God for the gift of my malleable soul and this POF journey that has brought me closer to Him.

He had a beautiful day at the park

Jo Clements

Jasper was born at 8.12am on 23 April 2010, one day over his due date. It was a long and arduous labour, but that didn't matter once he arrived. He was perfect. He looked nothing like we had expected – no sign of the dark features that we assumed he would inherit from his father. White blonde hair and eyebrows, and eyelashes so light they were barely there. Perfect.

On 25 May 2010 Jasper's father waved goodbye to him for the last time. He headed off to work overseas for just the one week. Jasper was 32 days old.

The following day, minus Dad, began as per usual. Jasper woke hungry and was duly fed, the day revolving around his feeding, nappy changing and sleeping times. At three we met with fellow mums and babies in a local park for coffee. He was sleepy, and in a moment of wanting to show Jasper off I woke him. It was, along with the last 32 days, one of the happiest days of my life.

The journey home through the park was broken by the demands of babies needing to be fed. It was a beautiful sunny day, and a stop under a tree to feed was no big ask. Jasper slept the rest of the way home. Unbeknown to me at the time, his life had already begun to slip away.

Here I have to pause. I am only able to tell this story in small pieces at a time. The day he died is still raw in my mind. I miss him and love him so much and am still coming to terms with his unexpected death. I want to tell this story because many are affected by similar circumstances. I've been able to take comfort in hearing the experiences of others: to hear how their grieving process is similar to mine and to have my range of feelings validated and normalised.

Having returned home, Japser peacefully sleeping in his pushchair, I took advantage of the downtime and put a few items away. However, within minutes of doing so, and while in another room, I heard Jasper gasping. By the time I reached him he was blue from head to toe. My first reaction was to put my finger in his mouth to clear what I hoped was just an obstruction. This didn't help, and the only thing I could think to do next was call an ambulance.

We were at the hospital within 15 minutes of the call – Jasper's colour revived from the oxygen the ambulance crew fed him. The hospital staff were ready for us and he was immediately seen by a team of paediatricians, specialists and nurses. My understanding of what went on for the next three hours is limited; what I understood at the time was that he was unable to breathe due to a vast amount of blood in his lungs.

I am eternally grateful to the ambulance crew, who stayed with me during the first hour while I waited for friends and family to arrive. I am eternally grateful to the nurses and the ambulance driver who helped me make calls to my husband, who was working in Romania, and to my family in New Zealand – particularly to my parents who had only left the UK two days beforehand.

What happened in those three hours is something I could never have been prepared for.

Jasper passed away at around 10pm on 26 May 2010. He was 33 days old. After a gruelling three hours a nurse, with a look of helplessness, came to tell me that they had to let him go; that they had been trying to resuscitate him for too long and his major organs were beginning to fail. This was the same nurse who, two hours earlier, had shed some light when

Jasper cried out; at that point she told me he was going to be okay and that I would get to hold him soon. Weeks later, she acknowledged that she felt bad for getting my hopes up.

The staff on duty that night did everything they possibly could to save him. There were nurses, who were not on his case, in the staffroom praying for him. There was nothing that anyone could do.

I felt, and still do, guilty about that night. I could barely look at my baby boy, who had tubes coming from his mouth and nose, was hooked up to machines making strange noises, and had a team of six or so people around him. I held and stroked his arm and gave him encouragement that one time he cried out. Most of the time I looked on from a distance, I felt helpless and scared, I was terrified to look at him. The doctor reassured me that they had given him medication so he would feel no pain. I'm not sure I would have made it through the night without the support of friends and family who were there with me at the hospital.

It hurts to recall this painful night. As Jasper's mum I had expectations that I should be able to protect him from all kinds of harm.

On the morning Jasper passed away he looked angelic. I later found out that the onset of what caused his death happened very rapidly, it started that afternoon.

Here is a link to my blog site: http://jasperatinylife.wordpress.com

His one and only birthday cake

Anne

Everything was going well with my third pregnancy, until I started to lose weight. So my husband Gilbert and I were pleased when the scheduled 18 - 20 week scan was coming up.

Monday arrived and Gilbert and I eagerly waited for the sonographer. He came, and found my placenta, my cervix and the baby's head. He then told us he could not see the baby well enough and needed to talk to his supervisor.

I turned to Gilbert and asked if he thought something was wrong. He confirmed my fears with a nod. Then we prayed. The supervisor arrived and stated that there were some grave concerns for our baby. In that second I thought *"oh no, they are going to tell me my baby is so deformed that I should abort and I will say no"*.

She took me aback stating *"your baby is dead"*.

How could that be? We had prayed, and waited and waited for this baby. We were over 12 weeks and I had no pain or bleeding so surely everything must be all right. Only last week I had felt the baby kick for the first time.

We stared at the screen, seeing a tiny head and knowing our baby was in heaven. The head of radiology arrived and said this was a very rare occurrence. He also said that there would be tests and that our midwife had been contacted. They asked what the 12-week scan had shown – we had not had one. I regret that now. All we could do was cry. We left, shell-shocked.

As soon as we arrived at my parents' house my mother knew something was wrong. Gilbert told our boys Eric, (five) and George (three), what had happened.

Next we had to tell Gilbert's family. During the car ride George asked why he couldn't hold the baby. I told him that Jesus wanted to hold him more. He seemed happy with that.

I was wondering if it was in some way my fault that baby had gone – should I have not picked up the boys so much, did I eat something? However, the next moment my midwife called and told me it was nothing I had done, this just happens sometimes. She briefly explained what my options were and said we could wait. However, I was eager to move on – not to feel like my baby's coffin.

I greeted my Mother in Love, Lily, with a hug and told her our devastating news. She was in total shock, she knew how long we had waited for this baby, and I was up to tissue 50! We called our friends and family with the news. My brother, a paramedic, mentioned how they often remove deceased babies. I was not ready for that. Everyone was shocked. After all, I had two healthy boys, two 'normal' pregnancies – why had this happened?

We went home, put the children to bed, had takeaways and talked. Later that evening my in-laws arrived with dessert, and two close friends came with flowers. It was good to talk. That night Gilbert and I prayed and discussed names. As we did not know baby's gender I was thinking of Angel but it did not fit quite right. *"Gabriel?"* Gilbert suggested. *"Perfect!"* So Gabriel it was.

The next day, Tuesday, we went to the hospital to discuss the big question – what next? When the doctor finally arrived he explained our two options: D&C (dilatation and curettage) or abortion pill – neither sounded good to me. Again Gilbert and I prayed. We decided on the abortion pill as it was less intrusive (we did want more children), and the doctor said we might be able to get hand and foot prints. I was excited, that was proof we really had a baby. I took the pill. The doctor informed us that I would be back in hospital on Thursday to deliver our baby – I was petrified. What would the baby look like? Did we want to see it?

We went to my in-laws' house to pick up the boys and ended up staying the night. It was wonderful to sit in a chair and listen to Gilbert's siblings talk, then to fall into bed. On Wednesday we went home, to be greeted by flowers and food. It was such a blessing to have others acknowledge that we were hurting.

By lunchtime I felt awful. I knew that something serious was going on when I nearly passed out. I looked at the information the hospital had given me, but was not sure what was happening. As my mum had her arm in a cast I called Lily. She came as soon as possible.

Only my two boys and I were home. I fed them lunch and nearly passed out again as the pain was so intense. I remember crouching on my hands and knees and my son asking *"what's wrong Mummy?"* I told him I was just working through some pain. He went back to eating. My younger son George needed help buttering his bun so I crawled over to help him.

I was so thankful when Lily arrived. I went to the bathroom and was stunned. I had just birthed my baby. I heard my eldest son Eric at the door asking if I was all right. I said *"yes"* and told him not to come in the bathroom but to get Grandma for mummy.

Lily was at the bathroom door with a shocked look on her face – there I was, standing holding who knows what? I knew it was the placenta but where was the baby? Lily got a bowl and we placed it into the cupboard so the boys would not see.

I called the hospital and they said I should come in, so I phoned my husband who was in a meeting. While waiting I looked at the information from the hospital. It said that just 0.9% of women miscarry at home after the pill, another rare occurrence.

When Gilbert phoned he was shocked. He met me at the hospital carrying our precious package. A nurse took a look and confirmed the baby was still in the sac and the placenta was intact. I felt relieved, mostly I think because I did not have to go through Thursday's labour. They cleaned baby and brought him to us in a box. We were afraid to look but did. He was definitely a boy, with perfectly formed eyes, nose, tongue – even though he was only 17 weeks.

I said to Gilbert *"he looks just like you"*. Everyone laughed. It felt good to laugh. We took photos, cried and prayed. We felt God's presence and peace. Then we said goodbye.

Next we needed to make more decisions. Did we want Gabriel to be tested? Did we want him returned to us? We decided yes to the testing but no we did not want him returned – where would we bury him? We knew he was already in Jesus' arms. They took blood tests and gave us a book with his hand and foot prints in it. Now I was ready to go home!

In the next few days Gilbert took the boys out so I had time to breathe, grieve and pray about where to next. What would we do to say farewell to Gabriel?

Gilbert and I felt it was important to acknowledge Gabriel's life. I had taken photos, including one of the boys hearing his heartbeat, and we felt we should make an album. So I set about collating all that I had and wrote a poem. The boys drew a picture each and Gilbert chose a song – *Blessed be the name of the Lord, He gives and takes away*. Sands sent us a birth certificate.

Day three was hard. I got the baby blues with no baby to cuddle. Instead I was hanging out washing and crying. A lady from church rang me to ask how I was doing – what a treasure! I also found it hard going from being pregnant to 'normal' in three days – I felt empty and lost.

My parents looked after the boys while Gilbert and I went away. This was a much-needed break. We were able to focus on Gabriel, our loss and our future. We spent time talking and just being together. We bought the album for the farewell. We had time to just 'be' as we both felt quite exhausted.

It was decided that the farewell would be at our house, and when we were on our way home I was thinking about all the work I had to do to make the house ready – windows to wash, the backyard to tidy, and what were we to do with the baby room? We had renovated to make enough room for the boys to sleep in one room. Now we had a spare one.

The next week was challenging. As I was so far along with my pregnancy, everyone knew. So each day there was a new group of people to tell. This was exhausting. One of the harder times was telling a friend who was due five days after I was. I told her mum and asked that she pass on the news. I cried. I knew how hard the news would be for her to hear. We attempted to get back to normal, whatever 'normal' was now, as we felt that was the way the boys would adapt best. They would talk about Gabriel in their play.

The album was a wonderful experience. As Gilbert was vacuuming and tidying for the farewell I was sorting and sticking. I would ask him what he thought of a page and he would offer suggestions. I can look at the album today and know it was something we did together.

The farewell was a positive time. My mother made him his one and only birthday cake – I cried! My friend gave me the blanket she had knitted for him – I cried! I had a display of all the things that reminded us of our little angel. My father-in-law read from the Bible and my father prayed. Our boys let off a powder blue balloon each to say goodbye. It was very special.

The weeks that followed were hard. Every time I saw a pregnant woman I would think that should be me but would then try to remember that God has a greater plan. We had to go to a party where several boy babies were. I felt isolated and alone but God brought along women with similar hurts and it was wonderful to talk to them.

Physically I was unsure of what to expect. I ended up with two infections and it took a fight of two and a half months before I got my first scan to find out if I was clear. This was also draining emotionally and mentally. As we had other issues going on at the time I imagined every little thing that came up was a big issue. I am sure everyone thought I was a bit strange, but it all felt huge.

I also felt as if I was playing catch-up. Several of my friends were expecting and now I was not – I felt hollow and flat. I found it very hard to get excited about anything, especially Christmas. My baby was due on 22 December.

Of course a lot of people told us we had to move on, keep living, that everything was for the best. My head knows that but someone needs to tell my heart. Someone asked me if my two boys were more precious now that I had lost one. My answer was no, they have always been precious to me.

As to more children, we do not know what the future holds but we know who holds the future. For now, I know I have birthed three children – two lovely rambunctious boys and one precious baby named Gabriel.

No apparent reason

Emily Campbell

My husband and I decided on our third wedding anniversary, in February 2006, to start trying for our first baby. At the end of April I did a home pregnancy test and got the good news that our baby was on its way. I was due on New Year's Eve, so decided on a midwife from the community hospital team as I discovered that it was very hard to find an independent midwife to deliver during the Christmas holidays.

My morning sickness was terrible from about seven weeks onwards. When I was 11 weeks pregnant my husband and I were out walking at the beach when I suddenly fainted face first in the sand. A passing ambulance stopped to offer assistance, and I ended up being admitted to hospital for fluids, monitoring, overnight observation and a scan.

Everything was fine with the baby, so we decided to let everyone know our good news rather than waiting for the 12-week scan the following week.

On Friday 14 July 2006, when I was 15 weeks and five days, I had some spotting and rang my midwife to ask if that was normal. She replied that it could be, and not to worry unless I had blood gushing down my legs. We were due to go away for the night with friends the next day, so we decided to keep to our plans since it was only a two-hour drive from home. As we were leaving the house on the Saturday morning (15 weeks and six days) I went to the toilet and found a large spot of fresh red blood in my knickers. I was excited about the night away, and thinking of the midwife's comments the day before. I decided not to worry too much.

However, when we arrived in Mangawhai, there was more bleeding so I decided to wear a pad. The bleeding continued throughout the day, and I confided in the friend that we were away with. At dinnertime I was concerned enough to ring my midwife again. As I was now out of Auckland, she told me to come and see her the next evening for a scan at the hospital, but still to not worry as many pregnant women experience bleeding.

A few hours passed and I was now dripping blood into the toilet every time I went to the loo – which was often as I was now getting very concerned. During one bathroom visit I felt a sudden gush of fluids into the toilet, which I later realised was my waters breaking. Again I phoned the midwife to tell her about the gush, and again she said that it may just be normal. By now I was starting to have some cramps as well.

Bedtime arrived, it was around midnight I suppose, and my cramps were worsening. My pad was soaked and I didn't have any more with me, so I wore one of my friend's son's nappies to bed. My husband fell asleep, but I lay awake with the pains worsening and becoming very regular and frequent.

At 1.10am on Sunday 16 July, I woke my husband up and told him I wanted to go home and to the hospital. I got up to go to the toilet and I felt the baby fall into the nappy and knew it was all over. I went into immediate shock, and my husband raced off to awaken our friend (she is a nurse) and call the midwife again, who advised calling 111, which he did.

Our friends came into my bedroom to comfort me, where I was lying on the bed in a pool of blood. The baby was still attached by the umbilical cord and was hanging between my legs, but my contractions had stopped and my cervix had clamped shut. An ambulance arrived – did the police, who had misheard the 111 call and thought that a 16-week-old baby had died rather than a 16-week miscarriage. I was put on oxygen and had an IV (intravenous) lure inserted. I was haemorrhaging and there was discussion of getting me airlifted to hospital, but it was eventually decided to continue to the hospital by road. I was lifted – bedding and all – into the waiting ambulance and taken to hospital. Midway we met up with another ambulance with an advanced paramedic on board, who assessed the situation and then followed us to the hospital to be on hand in case the bleeding worsened.

At around 3.30am we arrived at the A&E and I was again admitted to hospital. The baby was still attached by the umbilical cord and dangling between my legs and I was near hysterical with the trauma. My husband and I were both crying openly; I had never before, and have never since, seen him cry. At 4am I was finally given drugs to induce more contractions and deliver the placenta. I reacted violently to the drugs and started vomiting and needed a shot of anti-nausea medication.

The baby was taken away in a metal kidney bowl and cleaned up and returned to us in a little basket with a satin sheet. The A&E doctors and nurses were referring to 'the foetus' and the 'spontaneous abortion' but I was too upset to correct them and tell them how offensive that was. I asked them to find out what was wrong and why I had lost my baby, but they brushed me off and said it was 'only' my first miscarriage so there was nothing they could do for me. Everything appeared normal with the baby, who was the correct size and development for 16 weeks, and there was no apparent reason why I had miscarried.

I was moved to another ward for the night, and had a lovely nurse looking after me and following me to the toilet to look at all the clots and tissue that I was passing. She brought us information about the local crematorium and a tiny little knitted outfit, and arranged for the baby to be taken away to be cremated. In the meantime, he was left by my bedside in his little basket. We were never officially told the sex of the baby, but we think it was a boy. None of the doctors and nurses could definitively tell, and mercifully we were not sent to the Labour & Delivery ward for a 'professional' opinion.

We didn't dress the baby – the clothes were for premature babies and were still far too big for this tiny baby who was no longer than my hand. We never picked him up from the basket as he looked so fragile and vulnerable. Nor did we name him, mainly due to the uncertainty over the gender.

When morning finally arrived, and we still hadn't slept, we were anxious to get out of the hospital and go home to Auckland. We phoned our friends back in Mangawhai and arranged to be picked up from the hospital. I was in my pyjamas and bare feet, and had no camera or anything on me. It didn't occur to me to ask them to bring anything, so we haven't got any photos or keepsakes. We said our goodbyes to our baby as we left the hospital room. The next time we saw him was when we collected the ashes on the Friday of that same week.

What followed was a terrible time of grief. I cried many many tears. Having never lost anyone close to me before, I was overwhelmed by the intensity of the grief and how it could hit you like a truck when you least expected it. I had to tell my family, friends, workmates what had happened, and each time was like reliving a nightmare. Mostly though, I found it cathartic to talk about it, and have people acknowledge my loss and my emptiness.

My husband was wonderful, but he seemed to 'recover' a lot sooner than I did. But I know that, even now, it still hurts him to think of it, and he can't bear to scatter or plant the ashes as he likes having them with him in the house.

I visited my GP in the following weeks, and as well as prescribing sleeping pills for my insomnia and nightmares that had developed, he also arranged for numerous blood tests and an X-ray of my uterus being filled with dye, but no cause was ever found for my miscarriage.

My blood clotting levels were ever-so-slightly elevated, so for subsequent pregnancies I was on a low-dose aspirin, as the most likely explanation is that a blood clot formed in the placenta and caused it to break away from the uterine wall, thus suffocating the baby's air supply and inducing labour.

My midwife came and did a home visit the week after I lost the baby and we didn't even speak, she just sat in the lounge with me and watched me cry for half an hour before leaving again. I never saw or heard from her again, though about a month later an envelope arrived in the post with a brochure about miscarriage support. It is a very lonely time following a miscarriage, especially a second trimester loss, which falls in between regular miscarriage and stillbirth. Nothing is legally recognised, and I was never offered any counselling or support. I did speak to a workplace counsellor several times, and she highlighted the importance of recognising both the loss of the baby itself and also the physical trauma of the how and where it all took place.

On our due date of 31 December 2006 we released a balloon for our baby as we sat and watched the sun rise – unfortunately we were isolated out at the beach so there was no helium, and the balloon floated a few metres away and popped on a gorse bush. At that time I was eight weeks pregnant with pregnancy number two, and I'm pleased to say that we are now blessed with three lovely daughters, and we often think of the little boy that we never got to meet.

[211]

Reactions to my pregnancy

Amanda Whitehead

This story is written as if I am talking to my daughter about the time we had together.

In June 2009, Mummy was house-sitting for Mary and John. I was excited as they lived on a farm and it reminded me of my childhood. During the month, the sheep kept multiplying and I was worried as four sets of twins had appeared and some had had only one, and spring was not near yet. I kept wondering what was in the water.

July was a little sad as Lou, my adopted grandfather, passed away from cancer and I was honoured to be able to read a poem at his service. During the time of the funeral I had a funny inkling that something was different about me. I was more emotional and I just thought it was because of Lou's passing and my period being late. I took a pregnancy test on Friday 30 July. Wow, imagine my surprise, I was pregnant, you were growing inside me. Unfortunately, Daddy was not so impressed and decided to follow his own path.

As I think back now, I think that the water at the farm had some kind of pregnancy juice. I calculated the days and worked out that you were conceived on 25 June 2009 and due to be born on 17 March 2010. Now people are too scared to sleep in the bed at the farm in case they become pregnant!

Over the next eight months, our lives changed a lot. I had to try and find a new job, but was being knocked back because you were coming. I kept thinking to myself *"how could something so special and exciting be a problem for employers?"* It made me angry at how I was treated even though they couldn't say it, even though I knew you were exactly the reason. I held my head up high and kept going for interviews. Unfortunately I was unsuccessful.

During the eight months, I got prepared for you. I became very excited. I was going to hear 'Mum', and not just 'Miss'. I was going to be fully responsible for someone, not just caring for other people's children. Every time I went into a shop it was hard for me not to buy you something as it all looked so cute and maybe you might have needed that. I didn't buy clothes as I was unsure what sex you were. You had two baby showers, you lucky thing. You are loved by a lot of people.

During my pregnancy I was diagnosed with gestational diabetes so you had to be induced before 40 weeks. Friday 12 March came, and I was rung and told that you were not able to be born as there were no spare beds in the hospital. So I had a shower, washed my hair and straightened it nice so that you would see a beautiful Mummy when you were born. I went to sleep early thinking about the next day.

At 8.30am Saturday 13 March we were sitting in the waiting room, waiting for Gran to come. She arrived and we went into the pregnancy clinic.

During your labour, Gran and Aunty Barb were each holding Mummy's hands. Clare kept telling them to have a look, but they didn't. After a few more pushes, they couldn't stop themselves and they had to have a look at you being born. I remember saying to Aunty Barb, *"only take pics of the baby"*. *"Okay"* she laughed.

You were born at 3.09am on Sunday 14 March. Clare placed you straight onto my stomach and we looked straight at each other. You were so silent, just staring up at me. Then Gran cut your umbilical cord and you were away singing. *"What a set of lungs you have"* I thought. Mummy can't remember much after that, only a few bits and pieces and what I have read in the autopsy report. I'm sorry, Mummy was tired.

I remember looking at the clock and it was 4.17am. Clare was on the speaker calling *"Code Blue"* and then there was a large group of doctors and nurses in the room and they were trying to get you to breathe again. I was beside myself in shock. I did not know what to think. I remember the nurse saying that you were okay, you were breathing. I was reluctant to believe that as they kept putting the breathing machine on your face. I said *"why are you doing that then?"*

At about 11am we had a meeting and I didn't really know what was going on around me. All Mummy could think was *"what the hell happened?"* I didn't really listen at the meeting, I was still in shock.

After the meeting I couldn't sleep and everybody kept saying that I needed to. So I amused them all and went to my room and hopped into bed. All I kept thinking about was you. Everyone had gone home and I sneaked down and sat with you in the NICU (neonatal intensive care unit), all on my own. I just sat and looked at you, trying not to cry, trying to be brave.

The next 72 hours were a blur and all I wanted was to have you in my arms. Meeting after meeting was a haze and then I had you with me. Even after they took you off the life support I was not with it properly to know that you had passed, but you were with me. You were in front of me. I could see you.

I took you to Aunty Barb's house and you were cuddled by lots and lots of people who were waiting for you to arrive. I was happy that you were home. Seeing you made me very happy and I felt content in my heart.

None of Mummy's family came to see you, as death and bodies are not something that is acceptable to them.

After your funeral, it finally hit me that you were gone. My arms were heavy and I couldn't stop crying. I didn't want to be around anyone. The only picture that was in my mind was you. Counsellors, doctors and my midwife would talk to me about how this was a tragic accident. I thought about the medication that I had had during your birth, did that have an impact? Again they said *"no, nothing contributed to your loss"*. I just wanted answers, and all I want to say is *"Paige, why are you not here with Mummy? Why did you have to stop breathing?"*

Life now, for me, living without you being in my arms, is hard. I feel that society is not ready to hear about baby loss and how hard I am finding it to get back to reality. What is reality now? Life for me has changed and I can't believe how mean some people in society are. I tell the truth about you and people's ignorance hurts. I can't get employment because of it. I am going to try going to an interview and not mention you. Please don't think I don't care as I really do, but I just want to see people's reactions.

I really want to scream and yell at how society is, but then I may get labelled that I am not coping and be put on medication, which is wrong, but I want my voice heard. Why do I have to live with the reason you are not here is that you forgot to breathe.

I hate how 'supposed friends' say things like *"your babies are not here with you because you were not in the right relationship."* That hurts. It's mind boggling to me. It makes me think *"did my carelessness at falling pregnant have an impact on such a tragedy occurring"* and *"hell no it did not"*. I look at how many relationship break-ups there are and they still have their kids.

I live now with how people ask *"are you over it yet?"* or people who you would normally talk with who now just completely ignore me. I hate how I am treated now. It's like my tragedy has secluded me in society and made people talk about me behind my back. I want to say *"walk in my shoes because they are sore and I can't find a plaster that will mend it"*. I hate how people say *"time will heal"*. For me, it's still fresh and time is not healing. I use time as an anagram and I think of an 'item' that belonged to you, especially your Pooh Bear blanket which we snuggled in together.

I know that alcohol does not help me, and when drinking I have told people around me *"don't bring up Paige if you don't want to see my tears"*. What hurts is that people will say *"has she stopped the waterworks yet?"*

They say that tragedies bring out qualities in people that you have never seen before. I can't believe how my aunty and uncle have disowned me because I wanted you to meet your daddy. I did what was in my heart, and I know that you were happy seeing him at the hospital. Their grief is their own, but why did they treat me so bad because of my loss? How selfish I feel. I am stronger than that. I will not let them make me feel that I made wrong choices. They are two family members who are no longer in my life.

On 28 July 2010 I found out that I was pregnant again. I cried when I found out that a baby was growing inside of me. I was so shocked, but I wasn't sad, mainly scared. I was scared because I didn't want to lose this baby like I lost you. I slept with my arms over my belly every night. I tried not to think bad thoughts, but on 30 September I woke up and I was spotting. I went to the scan on my own as I didn't want to disappoint anyone.

I was distraught to find out that my pregnancy had ended. I could tell straight away as the baby should have been bigger than it was and I could not see a heartbeat. I named him Lucas Junior. I felt in my heart he was a boy.

Again, all the grief that I experienced with you came flooding back, twice as hard. I stayed away completely from people and just thought *"why me?"* I felt suicidal but was too scared to take the plunge. *"Why can't the clouds open and lift me up?"*

People ask me, *"would you die"* and I announce proudly, *"hell yes, then I would meet my children and my mum"*.

I have found now that I am not around my normal friends as much because I feel different and they make me feel angry with what they say to me. I wish that they would think before they speak. I have found that making new friends has been more beneficial as they have no real expectations of me because they don't know me.

I miss you and Lucas so much and I can't wait to meet you and your brother and see my Mum again. Please give her a big hug and kiss from Mummy. I love you my darling, Mummy always thinks about you.

Seasons

Clare Laing

My husband Russell and I have lost a total of four babies on our journey to parenthood. In that time, I have become acutely aware of the way the seasons punctuate our lives. As each new season arrives, I remember a baby that I was expecting.

Spring

Our first pregnancy was in spring 2008. The day before our wedding I took a test and was surprised but delighted to be pregnant. The night before I got married I was up until one in the morning reading books on pregnancy. I told just a couple of friends and one of them bought me little woollen singlets in preparation for my winter baby.

Sadly, just three days after our wedding, I miscarried that pregnancy. While I was disappointed, I read up a bit about miscarriage and realised that to have one miscarriage early in pregnancy is very common and that I would most likely not miscarry my next pregnancy. That information helped me a lot and I was eager to try again.

Summer

In January 2009 I got another positive test. I was cautiously optimistic. The summer was hot and intensified my pregnancy symptoms. On 13 March 2009 I miscarried a tiny but perfectly formed baby boy at 12 weeks five days. It seemed particularly cruel that I had to go through this difficult pregnancy and have no bundle of joy at the end.

It was a particularly traumatic miscarriage. I had a urine infection, which was largely asymptomatic until it entered my blood and I got urosepsis. It was a very unusual case, so unusual that I have had several medical professionals query my story until they read my notes.

Something I found particularly unhelpful was the number of people who said *"it wasn't meant to be"*. In my opinion, baby George was real and 'meant to be' except that his mother had the bad luck to get an awful infection. I doubt very much that anyone would say that to a mother whose child was killed in an accident.

In any case, summer had ended and so had my pregnancy dreams.

Winter

Autumn came and went as I dealt with the grief and also physically recovered from my experience of losing George. Towards the end of autumn I got another pregnancy test. It was a pleasant surprise as there were only six weeks between my miscarriage and new pregnancy.

Winter was long and hard. I had heavy bleeding early in the pregnancy due to a subchorionic haematoma (a clot that had formed alongside the placenta). I was monitored and told to rest. I was anxious and tense. I couldn't bear to lose this pregnancy.

With such a short gap between pregnancies it felt like a very long first trimester. Even when I reached that magical 12-week mark, I was still very nervous. I had lost a baby past that point, therefore I could lose another. Naively I focused on the 24-week mark where a premature baby could survive (since joining Sands I have realised that, while babies born at this gestation can survive, it doesn't necessarily mean they will).

But I got there, I got to 24 weeks.

Spring

Spring 2009, I enjoyed a brief hiatus from anxiety and sadness. The 20-week scan had been fine, my baby boy was small but I figured that some babies are. My husband and I both have birthdays in spring and we celebrated these, plus our first wedding anniversary, with a BBQ party.

We had accepted our previous losses and were looking forward to our future. There were so many exciting times to look forward to. My best friend was getting married in December and of course the birth of our son would top off summer.

On 13 November I went to my work as a secondary school teacher. The senior students were preparing to go on study leave and it was hard not to feel some of their excitement. But by midday that day my world came crashing down. I had been concerned about foetal movements and contacted my midwife. She sent me for a scan, which confirmed my worst nightmare. I was 28 weeks and six days pregnant and my baby had died.

Elliott James Laing was stillborn the next day at 16.53. He weighed 710 grams. A later autopsy revealed he had died from intrauterine growth restriction due to blood clots to the placenta. I had severe pre-eclampsia and hypertension.

Summer

Summer came but my baby didn't (at least not alive and healthy the way I had imagined). The summer was bright and sunny. I am grateful for my friends, who rallied around and invited me on holidays and organised events for me and my husband. While thoughts of Elliott always loomed it was nice to have at least some things to enjoy.

On other days, though, I wanted the sun to stop shining as it was so much in contrast to my dark, dark mood. Towards the end of summer (around Elliott's due date) two of the women in my neighbourhood had babies. One day I heard one screaming and, as I didn't realise this neighbour had been pregnant, I actually thought I was going mad. Another tactless neighbour made a point of confirming that there was a new baby in that house and she was gorgeous. She did this without even referring to Elliott and the fact that I had just lost a baby. Many people had said and done lovely things but that particular comment really upset me.

Winter

Winter came and with it another pregnancy. It was truly the worst few months of my life. For the entire pregnancy I was a nervous wreck. I struggled with insomnia, and every time I couldn't sleep I would worry about how that could affect the baby. In any case my worries were unnecessary, because at 11 weeks it was confirmed that the pregnancy has been a blighted ovum and the baby had stopped developing at about six weeks.

I entered a deep depression. Life just seemed so unfair. I had many friends expecting babies later that year and, while I can now feel happiness for them, at the time I felt angry and jealous.

Wasn't it supposed to be one in four pregnancies that ended in loss? Surely four out of four was unjust. My emotional recovery was stunted by the fact that the physical recovery from this miscarriage was long and drawn-out. I bled for two months before I finally had a D&C (dilatation and curettage).

I felt trapped in my life. Should I just give up? My losses were apparently unconnected so there was no medical reason not to try again. I felt in limbo, should I just pursue something else like a new job or further study?

I felt that, at nearly 36 years old, if I wanted a living child I couldn't afford to take a year off. It was all or nothing.

Spring

At the time of writing, spring has brought new hope for me. I am six weeks pregnant. I am fortunate to be having my pregnancy monitored by the Recurrent Pregnancy Loss Clinic. This monitoring has made a world of difference to my mental state. I have had 48-hour monitoring of my HCGs (human chorionic gonadotrophins) and they are rising nicely.

I am very hopeful that I might just be using those woollen singlets in June 2011.

SUPPORT ORGANISATIONS

The Compassionate Friends – offers support after the death of a child
Website: www.compassionatefriendsnz.netfirms.com
Phone: 03 439 5915

Fertility NZ – offers support and education for people with infertility challenges
Website: www.fertilitynz.org.nz
Email: support@fertilitynz.org.nz

Grief Relief – offers information and support for bereaved parents and families.
Note that this service is not free
Website: www.griefrelief.co.nz
Email: claire@griefrelief.co.nz
Phone: 04 970 1222

Karen Jefferson – qualified counsellor and bereavement support, offers support
and resources. Note that this service is not free
Website: www.bereavementsupport.co.nz
Email: bereavementsupport@xtra.co.nz
Phone: 03 343 3391

Miscarriage Support Auckland Inc – offers support and information to all
women who have experienced a pregnancy loss, particularly miscarriage
Website: www.miscarriagesupport.org.nz includes a page with a list of other
miscarriage support groups in New Zealand
Email: support@miscarriagesupport.org.nz
Support line: 09 378 4060 Office: 09 360 4034

NZ Early Menopause Support Group – offers support to women diagnosed
with premature ovarian failure, premature menopause or early menopause
Website:www.earlymenopause.org.nz
Email:nzem.info@nzord.org.nz

The New Zealand Multiple Birth Association – offers general support to parents
Website: www.multiples.org.nz
Email: info@multiples.org.nz
Phone: 0800 489 467

The Nurture Foundation for Reproductive Research – researches ways to predict and prevent reproductive problems
Website: www.nurture.org.nz
Email: admin@nurture.org.nz

PATHS – offers support to help with post-abortion trauma healing
Website: www.postabortionpaths.org.nz
Email: carolina@postabortionpaths.org.nz
Phone: 03 379 7710

PND – offers support to women and their families in Wellington with postnatal depression
Website: www.pnd.org.nz
Email: pnd.wellington@gmail.com
Phone: 04 472 3135 or 027 870 6853

Sands – offers support and information to parents, families and whanau following pregnancy, baby and infant loss no matter the gestation, age and circumstances. Most volunteers are also bereaved parents.
Website: www.sands.org.nz
Email: contact@sands.org.nz
Phone: refer to website for directory of Sands contacts throughout the country (under *Local Groups* page)

TABS – offers support to help with trauma and birth stress
Website: www.tabs.org.nz

Twin Loss New Zealand – offers support for loss of multiples at any stage in pregnancy or beyond
Website: www.twinloss.org.nz
Email: twinloss@xtra.co.nz

Victim Support – offers support to people coping with crime and trauma
Website: www.victimsupport.org.nz
Email: nationaloffice@victimsupport.org.nz
Phone: 0800 842 846

To suggest the inclusion of other organisations in this section please email jenny@babygone.com. Details may be included in any future reprints.